ACUPUNCTURE
AND ITS INDIAN ROOTS

DIETRICH KLÜBER

First Edition 1994
Lichtwortverlag, Kuddewörde

Design by

Matthias Klüber
Graphics Workshop
22958 Rotenbek

ISBN: 3-89811-033-8

Herstellung: Libri Books on Demand

ACKNOWLEDGEMENT

The author conveys thanks to his intimate Indian revered friends, Kirpal Singh and S. Divyanand, who gave the inspiration for this book and to so many Indian students including his daughter Melanie without whom this tremendous work apart from the normal profession would not have been accomplished.

CONTENTS

INTRODUCTION

Due to the initiative of S. Divyanand a German doctor is now presenting the old science of Acupuncture, knowing which one can treat many diseases without doing harm to the patient.

Acupuncture is derived from the Latin words ácus´ and ´punctura´ which means ´sharp´and ´pinching´. So Acupuncture is a science in which you prick or pinch with sharp instruments ,mostly needles. Acupuncture works with the least technical requirements one can imagine and no high expenses are needed. A doctor of Acupuncture can help often those who could not be helped by other methods of medical treatment.

In this Acupuncture course the student may first learn the theoretical part. The student must diligently learn many facts by heart before he can dare to start his practical career under the guidance of some experienced Acupuncturer. At a later time the knowledge given in these pages will be widened by more books, going more into the details of the practical facts and the exact way of doing Acupuncture by learning from example. The aim of this book is to enable the student of medicine to treat the patient first in an easy way with some kind of recipe-Acupuncture if the disease is not complicated , which truly speaking is not the real Acupuncture but only a way to it. But for the beginner it is a good way to start with. Furthermore the method of individual Acupuncture is brought before the eyes of the student eager of knowledge according to the traditional rules.

After the description of theory and practical science you will about the indications, contraindications and point combinations for the most common diseases, which may occur more often during your Acupuncture work here in India as far as I got to know.

At last you will have a list for the localisation of the most common points. You will be taught the course of the so-called channels or meridians and the pictures of those are also included in the back part of the book as well as some literature available in English, addresses of acupucture societies and a list for the first technical aids and instruments an Acupuncture doctor has to purchase in order to begin with his treatment. All this cannot teach you Acupuncture as a whole, as you need a practical guidance and bed-side teaching in order to be self-convinced of your knowledge.

THE HISTORY OF ACUPUNCTURE

Some thousand years ago the Chinese emperor Huang Ti gathered all doctors around him and ordered them to write down all their knowledge of medicine. At that time Acupuncture was a well-known method of treatment because you could and still can cure the diseases at the very root. The saying of that time was:

The best doctors prevent diseases
Ordinary doctors cure diseases and
Bad doctors treat diseases without curing them.

Nowadays this saying is not quite true anymore as diseases have become more common to mankind but the meaning behind these words should ever be remembered. Several centuries ago Acupuncture was well-known all over the world but when the Chinese empire began to decline, this medical art was almost forgotten. Only in the last few fifty years it has started again to spread in every direction when the western doctors got to know of the painstilling effect of the needles. Many demonstrations were given that even operations can be performed only with anaesthesia of Acupuncture. This convinced even the scholars. It is known to the author nor to the historical books what role India played at the time of birth of Acupuncture but Bharatha is said to be the origin of culture and so it is not unjust to suppose that China must have been only a province in the old worldwide empire before the battle of Mahabharata which inaugurated the

Iron Age. Acupuncture must have been known to its full extend already to this society which was not belonging to India or China but was governing much larger countries of the world all over.

Still nowadays in India cauterisation that means burning the skin plays a role in medical treatment, a sign, that Acupuncture was known here before very well, as cauterisation is one of the methods of acupuncure. In 1980 the author met a patient here India, who had this cauterisation at a famous Acupuncture point situated in the ear. I have to tell you that there is a special kind of Acupuncture called 'Ear-Acupuncure' which is a form of Acupuncture which is very difficult to perform without an electrical instrument for measuring the skin resistance because on the small place of the ear more than 120 points are situated and must be localized on the millimeter exact.

So this knowledge of cauterisation and Ear-Acupuncture must have been common in the old days, so that one can presume that there was also some method of recognizing these small Acupuncture points in the ear.

THE WESTERN WAY

Since start of this century many doctors brought the knowledge of Acupuncture to the West. Here this science was clothed into a Western scholastic way. The names of the Acupuncture points were brought into a systematic order numerating them so that each and every point who had a special name before got the sign of its channel and a number. Of course it had been very difficult for the students to learn all those names and thus the new order was much helpful. All these points are no real points nor holes in the skin, but aereas where the flow of energy could be influenced best. Especially the western doctors where interested in the effect of Acupuncture in anaesthesia because here they could see that this method was really working as it suppressed the pains occurring in operations.

Even new special forms of Acupuncture were developed. For example the Ear-Acupuncture by the French Dr. Nogier, the Mouth-Acupuncture by the German Dr. Gleditsch and the controlled Acupuncture Dr. Bahr, which I may explain to you in one of the following books for advanced Acupuncture. Dr. Voll, a German too, developed a testing method by which one can clearly see where and how Acupuncture can be worthwhile and which medicine may help the patient and which not.

And now I dare to say that the time has come to promote this technique in India so that it may come back again to its origin. I will do my part to achieve this aim and I wish to have many followers amongst you for this request. Already there is existing an Indian doctors Acupuncture society since about 5 years which has its headquarters in Delhi. I suggest that you join this society so that you have support and a meeting point in order to exchange ideas and experiences. In the appendix of this book I will give you the address.

WHY ACUPUNCTURE WORKS ?

Let us look for explanations for the working of Acupuncture. In modern times we find several kinds of explanation.

1. Reflexes:

We know that our body has many nerves that send signals to the spinal column and the brain when innervated and that move muscles later on. From the brain nerve impulses are send via the spinal cord to each and every part of the body. We also call this segmental innervation. If I strike on the patellar tendon on your knee the reflex is the moving of the lower leg if you want it or not.

The reflex explanation of Acupuncture says that if I put my needle into some special point the nerves under the skin get signals, signals that move up to the sinal cord in the brain and then suppress the pain center in the brain and manage that other signals are sent back in order to bring the body in order again so that diseases go away.

2. Activity of hormones

When we insert our needles in the skin of the patient we realize that the skin around the needle becomes red especially on the white skin of Europeans. This induced the scientists to suppose that certain hormones are released by the needle pricking and it was possible to find them increasing in the blood during Acupuncture. These hormones might be pain-killing, stimulating the circulation and perhaps also working as cortison but produced by the human body itself.

3. Energy transfer

The classical Chinese way of explanation is that the Acupuncture points are only doors to energy channels within the body, channels that cannot be seen with our physical eyes and are neither identical with nerves nor blood- nor lymphatic vessels. By closing or opening one door or the other of these channels we can bring the energy circulation in order if it is disturbed and let the flow of energy get harmonized. Disorder of energy brings diseases, by order health may come again.

We can also pump energy in these holes or extract it from them as you will see later. Of course our western scientists who always want to prove everything that one knows already, looked for proofs for the existence of these points too. French scientists injected a radioactive fluid in the points and showed with an electronic camera that the fluid spread exactly along these channels or meridians which the old scriptures had postulated. Injections in other parts of the body had this effect not at all.

Measuring the electrical skin resistance we find that all these points have a lower resistance than the skin around. So many acupuncturists are using this effect to find the point on the millimetre exact as the author is doing.

1966 Prof.Keller from Vienna found more blood vessels and nerves at those points than on other parts in histological examinations.

Every one of you can have your individual proof. If you touch the places shown on the Acupuncture charts with your fingertip you mostly either find a painful reaction, some knot below your finger or you fall with your fingertip into some hole or ditch on the smooth skin tissue.

Sometimes patients who come to your surgery say spontaneously that the pain is radiating from there through this part to that part of the body and if you look upon your chart of the meridians, the channels, you'll find that it is exactly this and that meridian. The best proof I know however is the wonder that Acupuncture works. The patient, painstricken, goes goes away with a happy heart and even if all other traditional and scientific treatments fail this may be of effect in so many cases.

THE BASIS OF YIN AND YANG

Chinese wise men classified nature in a dualistic way of either being Yin or Yang. If I translate it in Sanskrit terms everything in the universe is either Prakriti or Purusha. But at the same time every small part of prakriti has a very tiny essence of Purushu within it. This is well shown by the Chinese symbol of Yin and Yang:

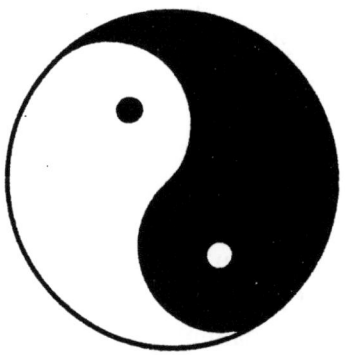

Now the Chinese people were mostly farmers and if a farmer works in the fields he always turns his back to the sun so that he does not have to look in it with his eyes. So the backpart of the body is full of sunlight; it is Yang. The other part, the face and stomach are more in the dark, the shadow and so they are of Yin quality. This dual thinking was transferred to everything existing in the world. So sun, fire and hatred are Yang as well as the moon, water and sorrow beeing Yin; only to mention a few examples. It is not so difficult to decide what else is Yin or

Yang or more similar to Prakriti or Purusha. If in a disease you find a state of fulness- Yang- you have to harmonize it by adding Yin or by reducing Yang and vice versa. This is the way how all Chinese philosophy and also your ayurvedic science which I revere most is working.

CHANNELS OF ENERGY

The old doctors found that the energy flow of Yin and Yang in our body follows certain roads or pathways which they called channels and which nowadays are called also meridians in the West. We devide them into Yin and Yang channels, seven each. There are some which are more Yang than the other Yang channels and there are some who are more Yin than the other Yin channels as you will understand quite well with the following picture of the farmer because some parts of the body get more sunlight than others.

Arms and legs can also be devided into Yang and Yin strips as you will see further. The back portion is still more Yang than the front portion. The middle portion has a middle stand .

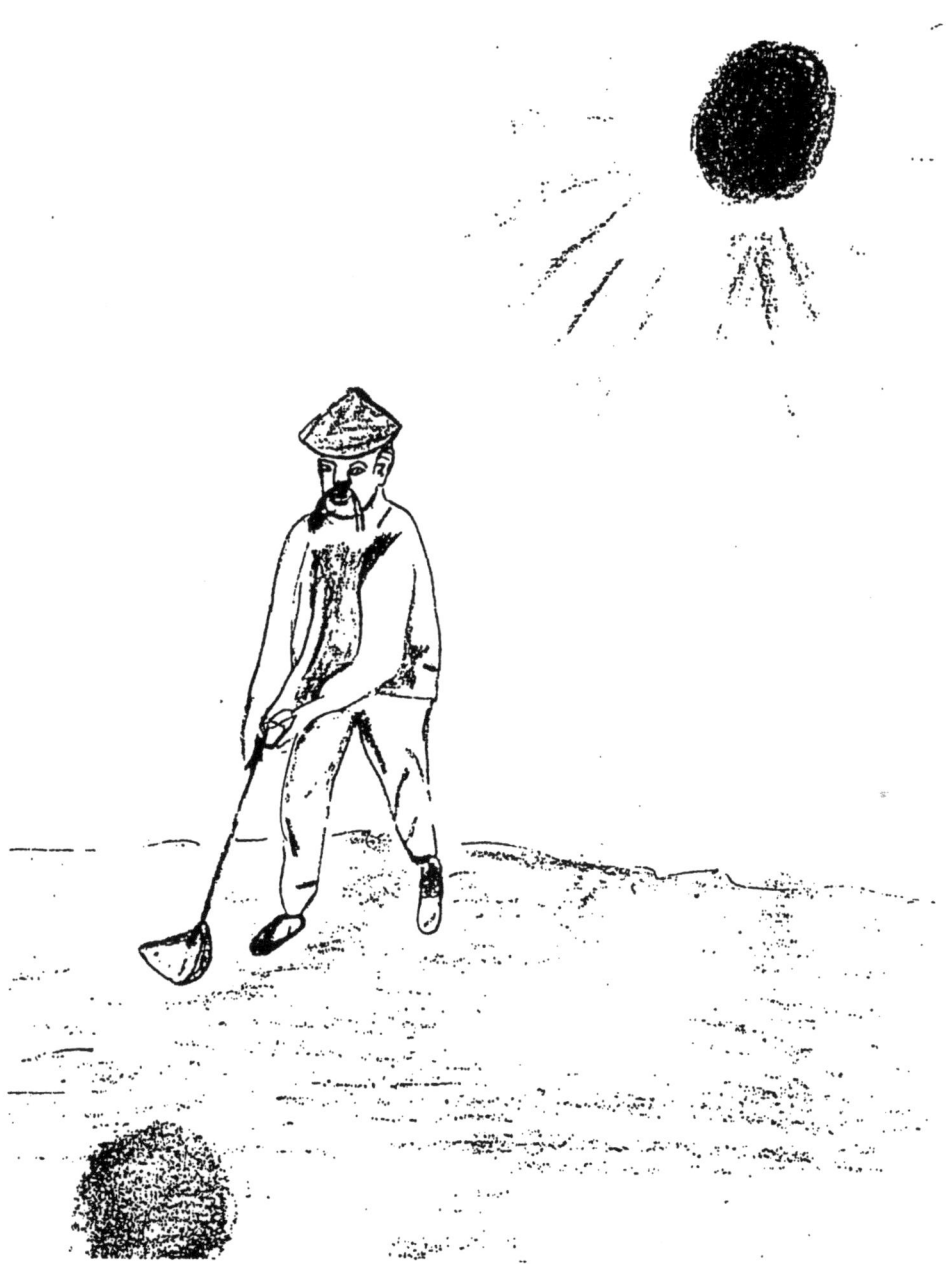

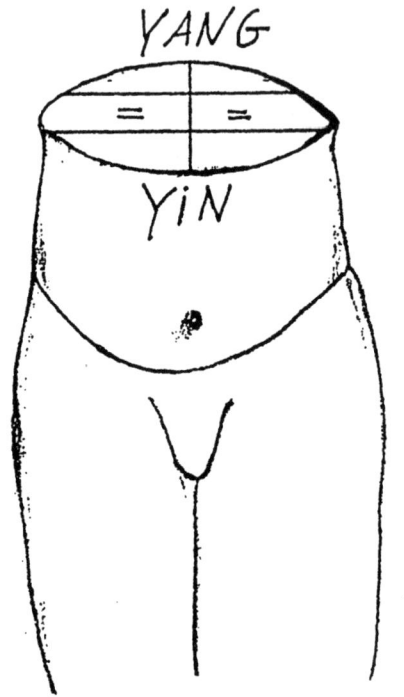

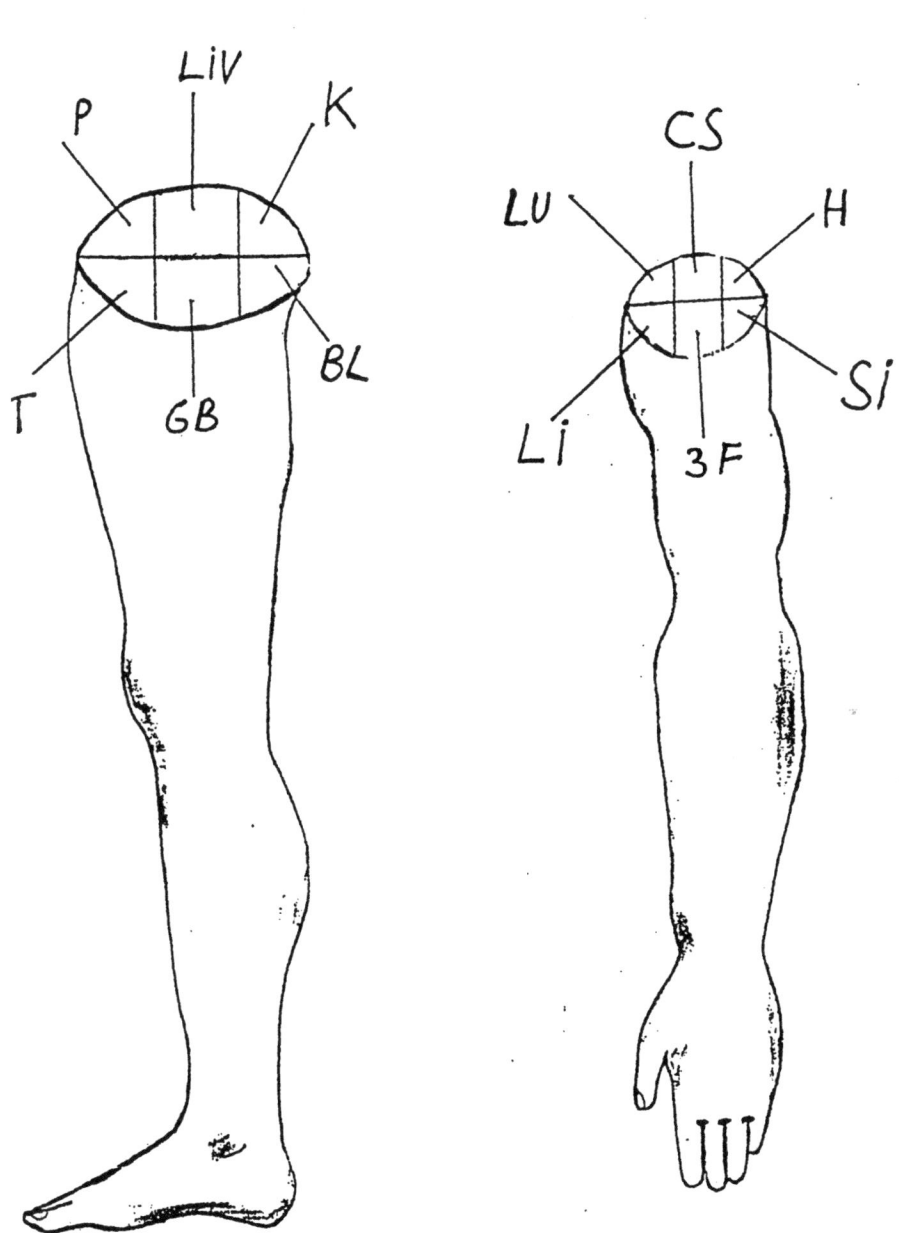

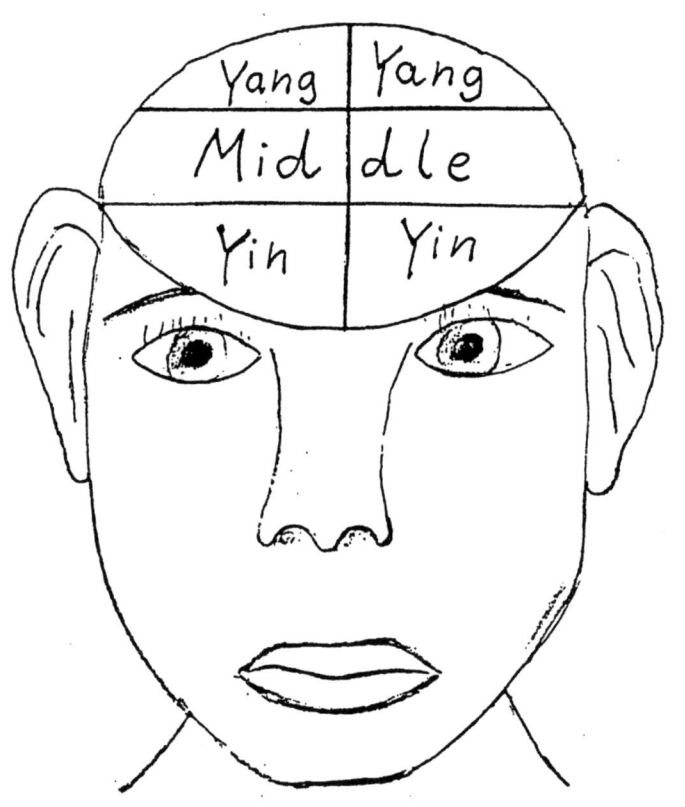

The channels have names which refer to their special functions.

The Yang channels	The Yin channels
Large Intestine (LI)	Lung (LU)
Stomach (ST)	Spleen (SP)
Three Fires or Triple Heater (3F)	Circulation/Sexuality (CS)
Gallbladder (GB)	Liver (LIV)
Small Intestine (SI)	Heart (H)
Bladder (BL)	Kidney (K)
Director Vessel (DV)	Conception Vessel (CV)

POINT BY POINT

As I told you before there are holes or points of Acupuncture and every channel has several important points that a student of Acupuncture has to learn. The channels either start or end at hand or feet. The other end is the starting point of the following channel as we will see later. These points are the means how the doctor can influence the body energy giving more Yang or Ying impulses to his patient.

On the human body you can find more than 800 such points. 360 were known to the Chinese. The others were found during the last decades by more exact methods. For the special part of ear Acupuncture we have already more than 120 points.

For a doctor in Acupuncture it is enough to know the site of 100 to 200 points with which he can achieve almost everything he wants. Every doctor has his personal points which he prefers, but all can be useful. Some special points which we will discuss later on more precisely everyone should know. The beginner can also do wonderful work with only 60 points. Those we will mention in the appendix of this book.

THE FIVE ELEMENTS

Chinese philosophy has much similarity to the old Indian which again underlines my thoughts that in olden days those regions had only one culture. As in Ayurveda Chinese doctors know of the existence of five elements. They just give them varying names. For the discussion of diseases it is worthwhile to know the significance of these elements,in order to find the best treatment. This is the case in Acupuncture too. In China they had the following five elements. In brackets I give the terms for them in ayurvedic science:

Metal (Vayu)
Water   (Jala)
Wood (Akash)
Fire   (Agni)
Earth (Prithvi)

By the following system you can understand how each element can be influenced by the different parts of the other elements. Each element occupies two Acupuncture channels; Fire four of them.

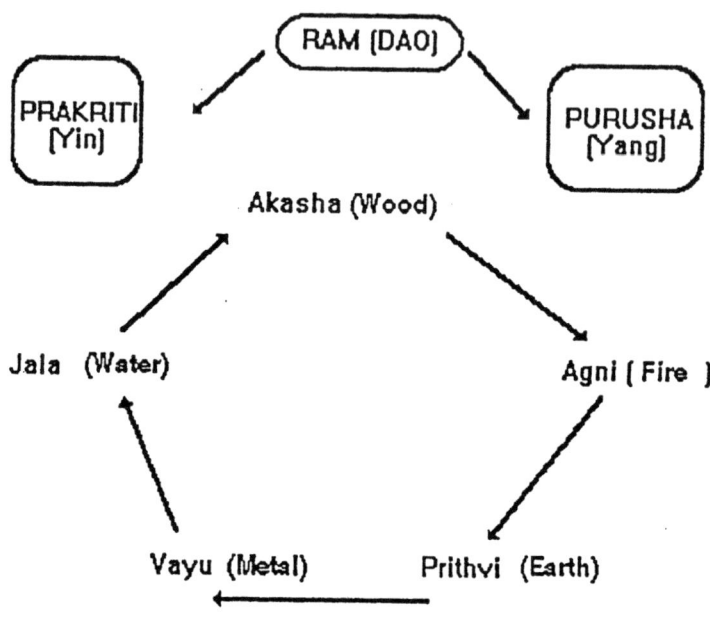

Wood occupies Liver and Gallbladder,
Fire occupies Heart, Small Intestine,
Circulation/Sexuality and Three Fires,
Earth occupies Spleen and Stomach,
Metal occuopies Lung and Large Intestine and
Water occupies Kidney and Bladder.

It is important to know that the elements have interconnections of multiply kind. First there is the promotion relation. Water promotes wood because wood grows by water. Wood promotes Fire because fire needs wood for burning. Fire promotes Earth because ashes go into earth again and give substance to the soil. Earth promotes Metal, because you get the metal in condensed form back from the earth again. Metal promotes Water because metal when heated gets into a water like fluid form.

The second relation is an interacting and overacting relation. For example: Water destroys fire. Wood consumes earth .Fire melts metal. Earth dams water. Metal is used to seperate wood with an axe.

The third is a counteracting relation. Now let us see what this means. Water can overcome earth by washing it away as one could see some time ago in Bangladesh. Metal can overcome fire by building a fence that is protecting us from fire. Earth can overcome wood by eating it up until it is rotten. Fire can overcome water if it is so strong that water changes to vapour. Wood can overcome metal if it is very hard, the axe gets broken. Thus the channels can also influence each other in the same three different ways.

THE CIRCLE OF ENERGY

From the above relations between the elements results the circulation of the energy within the twelve channels. This circulation is bound to time so that every channel has its maximum activity during two hours of the day.

Thus it is understandable why certain patients feel their suffering at some fixed hours of the day and it means that the Acupuncturer has to add energy, has to tonify or to lessen those channels or vice versa the opposite ones. It is for example very common that patients of asthma awake in the early morning between 3 and 5 a.m. with cough. The lung channel has in its maximum time not enough energy to make the damaged lung work properly. Those patients may also have difficulty between 3 and 5 p.m. because now again the lung channel has not enough energy due to its minimal working level. This would mean that we have to tonify the lung channel. The right time for doing it is naturally the time between 3 and 5 a.m.

Let me tell you the times of the channels now. I will tell you the maximum times of each channels. You will find the minimum times just by calculating twelve hours later. Please note the abbreviations already known to you.! With that you get a socalled organclock as the following picture is showing.

H:	11 a.m.-1.p.m.
SI:	1-3 p.m.
Bl:	3-5 p.m.
K:	5-7 p.m.
CS	:7-9 p.m.
3F:	9-11 p.m.
GB:	11 p.m.-1 a.m.
LIV:	1-3 a.m.
LU:	3-5 a.m.
LI:	5-7 a.m.
ST:	7-9 a.m.
SP:	9-11 a.m.

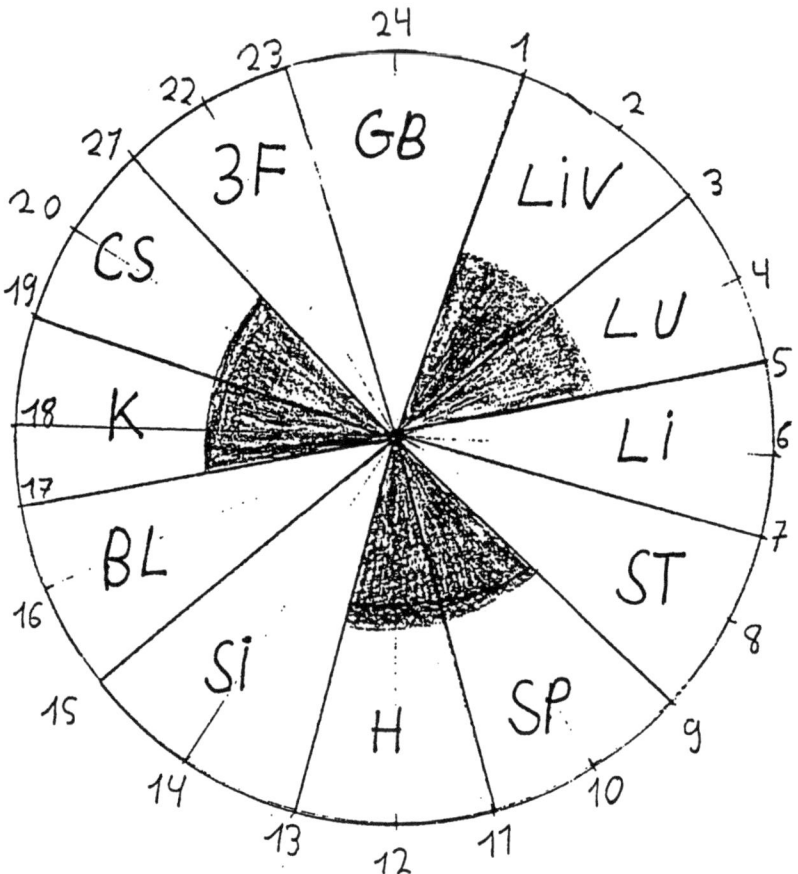

If you could follow till now you realized that two channels are missing, CV and DV. Easy as it is those two have the function to receive energy from above that means God or the Overself and to distribute it where it is needed respectively. Again I remember Ida and Pingala, the two channels that make their way round Sushumna, the central channel. Dont you find the relation to the Indian system of Patanjali Yoga ?

Referring again to the circle of energy you may have a look to the human body, the way the channels are taking on its surface. You will find that it is a nice constructed pathway from a Yang to a Yin channel at the same hand then coming back to the body center and here going down by a Yin channel again to the legs. Coming back again to the center by a Yang channel and so on and so on. Nature has made an excellent instrument.

Lung is the first channel, a Yin channel. It starts at the shoulder on the front, goes on the front of the arm just to the thumb. There the energy flown over into the

Large Intestine channel. The LI channel starts at the tip of the second finger on the outside, going up on the outside of the arm, turning to the outside of the shoulder then arriving on the neck and reaching and ending crosswords on the nose. Now the

Stomach channel starts.Below the middle of the eye it starts and courses in a U-turn to the temple .On the cheek the external branch runs downwards along the throat to the shoulder The channel follows the mamillary line along the thorax to the abdomen and lateral to the midline. It continues on the anterior side of the thigh to the lateral side of the knee and the lateral

29

border of the tibia to the back of the foot. The channel ends at the lateral corner of the second toe nail. Now energy jumps over from Yang to Yin and

Spleen channel starts. It starts on the medial side of the great toe nail, runs on the medial side of the foot to the medial side of the leg and along here to the lateral side of the abdomen. It jumps from here to lateral and upper side of the chest, then turns downward and in a lateral direction to end at the axillary line in the sixth intercostal space. Now the energy is going downward again within the

Heart channel. It decends from the axilla along the medial and ulnar side of the arm to the palm and ends on the radial side of the small finger at the nail corner. Now it is time to switch over again from Yin to Yang and

Small Intestine channel starts. It makes its course from the lateral nail corner of the small finger and passes upwards along the dorsal side of the arm to the dorsal side of the shoulder. The channel runs along the shoulder in a zigzag line and continues on the outer side of the neck to the cheek and the ear. Now it is time to get down again and

Bladder channel starts. It starts at the inner side of the eye and ascends first parallel to the midline over the forehead to the neck. At the neck the channel devides into two branches. The more important inner branch descends lateral and parallel along the midline 1 1/2 finger width to the forth sacral foramen where it turns backward to the first sacral foramen and then continues downward to the dorsal side of the thigh to the hollow of the knee to connect with its outer branch again. From the knee the channel descends along the dorsal side of the leg to the outer aspect of the foot and ends at the outer corner of the little toe nail. And now it is time to switch over from Yang and Yin and

Kidney channel starts below the foot palm running on the inner side of the leg to the abdomen where the channel is located half fingers width lateral to the midline. In the chest area the distance is 3 fingers width. The channel ends below the depression of the clavicle. Now we have to go down again and the channel of

Circulation/Sexuality starts lateral of the mamilla, then passes to the axilla, descending along the medial aspect of the arm to end at the tip of the middle finger palmside. Now energy switches over from Yin to Yang and the

3-Fires channels starts making its way up. It starts on the outer side of the nailcorner of the ring finger, ascends along the dorsal side of the arm to the shoulder, circles around the auricle and runs to the outer side of the eyebrow. In order to come down again the

Gallbladder channel starts. It originates on the outer side of the eye and runs down to the ear, circling around it and reaching the occipital region. From here the channel runs back to the forehead and then returns back parallel to the midline to the neck passing further along the shoulder to the side of chest, then descending on the outer side of the trunk and abdomen, the leg and foot where it runs around the outer ankle and ends on the fourth toe. Here energy switches from Yang to Yin and

Liver channel starts upward again. It starts on the great toe along the inner side of the leg and thigh to the genitalia then ascends on the abdomen to end at the lateral chest wall in the sixth intercostal space below the mamilla. Now we have ended our tour and Lung channel is starting again.

To describe the other two channels we have to mention that

Director Vessel starts at the Os coggygis, passes upward along the backside midline to the neck , runs along the midline on the face to the forehead and nose to end below the upper lip on the mouth. Here Yin is changing to Yang and

Conception Vessel starts. But it is better to say it ends here because its starting point is the perineum ascending along the frontal midline upon stomach and thorax and ending on the chin below the mouth.

Out of the flow of the energy as I have just described and the three interrelations of the elements follow the

ACUPUNCTURE RULES

Let me first describe the rule of

Mother and Son

The first meridian is the mother of the following. The following is the son of the one channel before. For example, LU is mother of LI and BL is son of SI. The practical importance for the therapy is that in order to tonify the son channel if it has not enough energy one should also tonify the mother so that the mother can give more to the son too. If you want to diminish the energy of a channel you can also decrease the energy of its mother channel so that the son cannot get too much from its mother in turn. Very easy isnt it? How one can stimulate or diminish the channel energy you will get to know later. The second rule is the rule of

Husband and Wife

It is combined with the classical pulse diagnosis which I find is purely a Chinese way of diagnosis as in the old books of Ayurveda like Caraka-Samhite you will not find mentioning so many qualities of pulse diagnosis as are taught today. But you will see that the diagnosis of pulse had much more importance than it has nowadays in the Western medical science. But the pulse diagnosis may have its value if it works in the hands of a very long trained practitioner. Otherwise it is very difficult to interprete and to differentiate between the qualities of the pulse. This you will have to learn in many years of experience.

But let us come back again to the rule of Husband and Wife. Chinese doctors found the channels beeing reflected in the different layers of pulse positions. There are two different layers and three positions where you feel the pulse at the wrist.

The layers are the deep or the surface layer. The positions are distal, proximal and medium. Medium position is situated at the inner side of the wrist near the hight of the bone you easily feel there. Let me tell you that for the present it is sufficient to know where the different meridians can be felt because from this location the rule of Husband and Wife originates. Let us take the first position which is the distal one.

On the right hand on the surface layer you will feel LI. On the deep layer LU. On the left side you feel on the surface layer SI and on the deep H.

The second position in the midth: On the surface layer on the right side you find ST and on the deep SP. On the left side superficially GB and in the deep LIV.

The proximal, the third position: here you can find on the right surface layer 3F and in the deep CS. Left on the surface BL and in the deep K.

If you compare the meridians on the right and left sides respectively and look to the interrelations on the same position at the same layer you will find the rule of Husband and Wife. That means: if you want to stimulate the husband you have to reduce wife as both are in opposition to each other as the married ones amongst you may agree to. If you want to reduce the husband channel you have to stimulate or tonify the wife

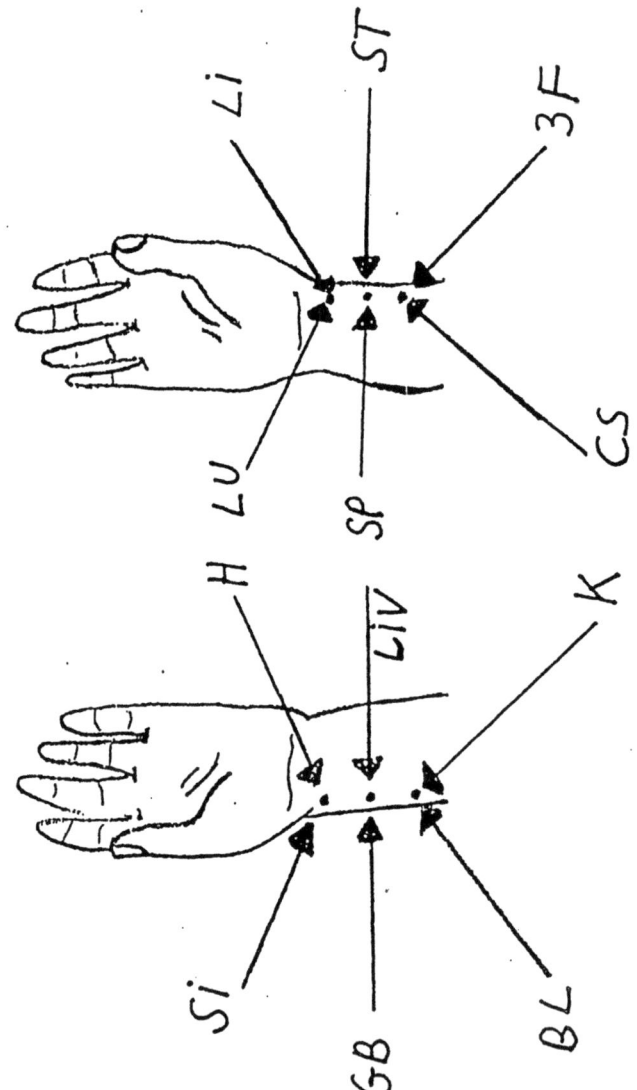

Now I will give you a list of the pairs of husband and wife:

WIFE	HUSBAND
LI	SI
LU	H
ST	GB
SP	LIV
3F	B
CS	K

The technique of pulse diagnose you have to learn from your ayurvedic teachers. They will inform you more exactly about it than I can do in this lecture. Next comes the rule of

Midday and Midnight

This rule we had already touched upon when we were learning about the energy clock. Those channels who are 12 hours in opposition to each other for those you have to perform the same procedure as under the rule of Husband and Wife. For example. If you stimulated H(Yin) the opposite channel GB (Yang) will be reduced. For this have a look again on the organ clock please.

The Rule of Up and Down or Yin-Yin or Yang-Yang Rule

As we have seen, there exist channels on the body which are either Yin or Yang or also in between, if they have some Yin part but the Yin Part is stronger and vice versa. In order to see how this Yin-Yin divison works, please remember the farmer working in his field standing over his crops and the sun shining on him from behind. His arms and legs are downwards. So now there exists a borderline between the hanging arm and the standing leg just in between, so that it separates hand and leg in two parts, one left and one right one.

Then there are more divisions. They are going from right and left and are separating arm and leg again in three parts right and left, one front part, one middle part and one back part. So now we have six different parts in hands and legs and they correspond to each other according to the amount of light they get by the sun shining from behind. You can understand it better with the picture already shown.

Now in each of these six longitudinal parts one channel is running and the channels in the respectively two corresponding parts of the six are combined and this is the Up and Down Rule. So I will now tell you the channels which are combined with each other.

On the outer side on the most backlying part of arms and legs are SI and BL, being Yang channels.

Again the most backlying part but on the inner side of arms and legs are the channels of H and K respectively being Yin channels.

On the inside middle part are CS and LIV, being of Yin quality, On the outside middle parts are 3 F and GB beeing of Yang quality.
The inner front part is belonging to LU and SP channel, beeing Yin, The outer front parts are concerned with LI and ST being Yang.

The outer front part has less Yang than the middle, the middle has less Yang than the back part.

On the inner Side it is vice versa.
The front part has more Yin than the middle part and the middle part has more Yin than the back part. This is as it is with the rule of Up and Down The next rule is called

Inside-Outside or Yin-Yang Rule

That means that the channels which are situated either on leg or on the arms on the same back, middle or front parts, are coupled with each other. By this you get six couples:

H and SI	(back part hand)
K and BL	(back part leg)
CS and 3F	(middle part arm)
LIV and GB	(middle part leg)
LU and LI	(front part arm)
SP and ST	(front part leg)

So the rule is in both cases that if in one part the pain or disease is situated on the course of one channel, you look for its coupled channel and choose some point on this one also

THE FIVE STEPS TO SUCCESS

The first step: How to find the right channel.

With right channel I mean the channel that is affected. You find the affected channel directly if you look to the place where the pain or dysfunction is situated. This channel which has its course through that place of the body is the affected channel and should be treated foremost. Indirectly you find the affected channel in chronic, complicated or inner diseases if you watch the function of the inner organ that is disturbed and think about which circle of function for which always one channels is standing, is disturbed.

The second step refers to the question how the disease could fall on the patient, whether his complaints have come from cold or hot, whether they where started after humidity or dryness or wind.

These are the outer influences.
Cold may affect K and BL, humidity may affect SP or ST, Hot may affect H or SI, Dryness may affect LU or LI, Wind may affect LIV or GB.

The inner influences are fear, sorrow, happiness, sadness and anger. Fear may affect K and BL, Sorrow SP and ST, Happiness H and SI, sadness LU and LI, anger may affect LIV or GB.

The third step is the question whether the patient or the disease are a type of weakness or fullness. Weakness has to be treated with near-by points and not so much stimulation. Fullness has to be treated with much stimulation and far-off points.

The fourth step. In the fourth step you ask which points of the affected channels are the most effective points. For this question you have to consider all the Acupuncture rules I have mentioned under this heading. But you should also consider that a point that is recommended may have different and multiply effects. So you can get the best combination with a few needles if you combine the effects of special points.

The fifth step. The question is now with which kind of stimulation you will be treating according to the root of the disease and according to the type of the patient. If the disease has come from coldness or humidity or wind or the patient or the disease has a type of weakness symptom then the stimulation will be needling,heating, treating with warmth and fleecing. If the type of the disease is one of fullness, if the root for the disease may be hot or dryness or the patient is of a fullness type, then you treat with needles and with bleeding.

POINT CATEGORIES

Among the more than 700 points on the meridians there are some classes of points which are most useful and you should know them exactly if you want to progress in Acupuncture:

Tonifying Points

Each channel has a tonifying point by which it can be stimulated more quickly. You can support the stimulating effect

if you use a golden needle

if you turn the needle clockwise when inserting it or

take it out quickly or

if you use Moxa (herbs of Artemisia vulgaris) or

give a little heating to the needle the tinder.

Sedation Points

Each channel has a point by which its energy can be reduced better than with another of its points. To make it easier you can use a silver needle or

turn the needle counterclockwise or

take it out slowly

Agreement Points

Each channel has an agreement point which is always situated on the Bladder Channel near the spine. The kind of measurement by which you will find the points will be explained later. The agreement points are mostly used in chronic diseases and respond to the segmental innervation of the body quite well.

Fountain Points

The Fountain points are used in combination with the Agreement Points or in combination with the Tonifying or the Sedation Points. They work as catalyst for these three groups and are thus very important as they fortify the result of them. Of course they can also be used alone.

Passage Points

The Passage points are the links between the channels that follow each other in the energy circle as are the Fountain points as well. For example LIV and GB are such interactive channels. LIV is Yin, GB Yang. By using the Passage Points you achieve an energy exchange between the two. If one has too much or too little both will have the same amount of enery at the end. By this method you can save needles as you dont have to reduce one and stimulate the other channel. You only use one needle at the Passage Point.

Alarm Points

The Alarm points are either situated on the Conception Vessel or the channel itself. They are used for acute diseases and may also be painful spontaneously if the respected channel is affected.

Cardinal Points

Cardinal Points should only be used by experienced doctors as they are able to shift large heaps of energy in a very short time. They are the sluice keepers that have to be handles with great care lest either you may provoke a flood or a dryness in the healthy channels.

Reunion Points

The Reunion Points are the crossings of several channels. Here you can also save many needles by using them. Especially if they are painful you should always take them into your program.

Lower Points

Only the Yang channels have such Lower Points. That means only the organs of ST, LI and SI, BL , GB and 3F.
Lower Points are situated on the legs and are used for acute diseases too.

THE TABLE OF POINT CLASSES

CHANNEL	Toni-ficatio n Point	Seda-tion Point	Agree ment Point	Fount ain Point	Pas-sage Point	Alarm Point	Car-dinal Point	Lower Point
LU	LU9	LU5	BL13	LU9	LU7	LU1	L7	
LI	LI11	LI2	BL25	LI4	LI6	ST25		ST37
ST	ST41	ST45	BL21	ST42	ST40	CV12		ST36
SP	SP2	SP5	BL20	SP3	SP4	LIV13	SP4	
H	H9	H7	BL15	H7	H5	CV14		
SI	SI3	SI8	BL27	SI4	SI7	CV4	SI3	ST39
BL	BL67	BL65	BL28	BL64	BL58	CV3	BL62	BL54
K	K7	K1	BL23	K3	K4	GB25	K6	
CS	CS9	CS7	BL14	CS7	CS6	CV17	CS6	
3F	3F3	3F10	BL22	3F4	3F5	CV5	3F5	BL53
GB	GB43	GB38	BL19	GB40	GB37	GB24	GB41	GB34
LIV	LIV9	LIV2	BL18	LIV3	LIV6	LIV 14		

Further some other groups of points can be mentioned:

Six Important distal points

LI   4 for the region of face, neck, sensory organs
LU 7 for neck and lung
CS 6 for the epigastrium and the front of the chest
ST 36 for the organs of the abdomen
BL 40 for the lower back and urogenital organs
SP   6 for pelvic organs and perineum

Other special points with the same effect are points with

Analgesic effect :	LI 4,ST 44,ST 43
Tonifying effect :	K6, K8, ST 36, SP 6
Sedative effect :	DV 20, Extrapoint 6, H 7 , BL 62
Homoeostatic effect:	LI 11, SP 6,ST 36
Immunenhancing:	LI 11, DV 14, DV 13
Influencial Points:	Point for storage organs LIV 13 Point for hollow organs K 12
Respiratory system:	K 17
Blood:	BL 17
Bone:	BL 11
Bonemarrow:	GB 39
Muscles+Tendons:	GB 34
Vascular System :	LU 9

All the mentioned points will be listed in the appendix with their exact location.

CHINESE REFERENCES

For diagnose it may be important for you to know the following list of references:

Yin organ	LIV	H	SP	LU	K
Yang organ	GB	SI	ST	LI	BL
Colour showing disease	Green	Red	Yellow	White	Black
Worse by	Wind, sour taste	Heat, Bitter	Humidity, Sweet	Dryness Hot	Coldness, Salty
Diet	Salty	Sour	Bitter	Sweet	Hot
Sense Organ	Eyes	Tongue	Lips	Nose	Ear
Body part	Nails	Face	Lips	Hairs	Hair
Affected	Tendon	Blood	Muscle	Skin	Bone
Mind	Rage	Happy	Greedy	Sorrow	Fear

Thus you have hints as well how to put the diagnosis and which channels may be affected. You can compare it again with your concept of Ayurveda which is not always with the same references. But you can combine them so that it fits for both systems. Ask me for special explanations in this respect.

HOW TO BE CORRECT UP TO THE POINT

A. The method of touching

Either the points are very sensible if the patient is very sick and has a deficiency or surplus of energy in the channel where the point is situated. By fingertouch you find them either smoother than the skin around or prominent as a little hill.

B. The method of measuring

Knowing the site of the points approximately by the measurement or Cun you can find them easily referring to prominent bone structures or other known points. Cun is an individual measure. 1 Cun is the width of the thumb or the length of the middle bone of the second finger of the patient. In Acupuncture the measurement is always given in Cun . For this purpose you can construct a Cun-Meter. How it is constructed, you can see on the next picture

Cunmeter

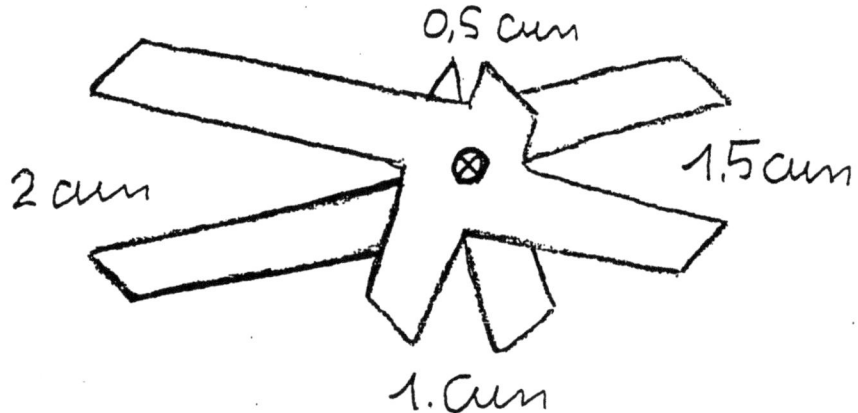

0,5 cun

2 cun

1,5 cun

1. Cun

Common Cun-Measures are the following:

1	Cun	Width of the thumb
1,5 Cun		Width from second to third finger on their basis
2	Cun	Width from the first to half of fourth finger
3	Cun	Width from second to fifth finger at their basis.
5	Cun	Distance from navel to Os Pubis
6	Cun	Width of the front without hair
8	Cun	Distance between the 2 nipples or distance from sternum's end to the navel
9	Cun	Distance between axillary fold and transverse crease of the elbow
12 Cun		Distance from transverse crease of the elbow to the wrist
16 Cun		Distance between middle of the Patella and the tip of the outer Ankle
19 Cun		Distance between greater Trochanter and middle of the Patella

C. The measurement with electric instruments

With instrument that measure the electric resistance of the skin you find the points as they all have a lower skin resistance. But you have to know the approximate site of the point at least lest you search for it at a far off place.

METHODS OF THERAPY

Needles are the best working instruments for Acupuncture. You should never do without them. Whether there is much advantage in using silver or golden needles there are much discussions. I think that it is not so much important, not only because these materials are much costly but also as you can stimulate or reduce the energy by using the special points or other methods. If you have steel needles which get not rusty, which are neither too long nor too short, and neither too thick nor too thin but always sharp at the tip you have everything you need besides your intelligence and patience.

The oldest form of Acupuncture must have been the **rubbing or massage** of the afflicted aerier. This can also be done by the patient himself. But in fact it only helps for a short time and will not fully cure the disease.

Moxa and cauterisation as explained before can performed with special Moxa cigars which are held over the points burning or by holding a tinder at the top of needle or by burning Moxa on the plate of special needles. With this you achieve an intense tonification of the afflicted channel. Cauterisation is a method that I do not like very much if it is performed with a hot iron as you have to burn the patients skin. It hurts, may cause infections, is brutal, leaves ever-staying signs and can be replaced by normal needles easily if you know your art of Acupuncture.

Electric stimulation of needles or with a pen of an electric instrument with a relatively low intensity of current and upto 200 Hz can be useful in acute diseases and pains or if some limb is paralysed. Often small children are much thankful for such a treatment which makes no pain at all if used without needles.

Here I want to mention the use of a **Laser Beam** too but I dont lay much stress upon it as the reaction does not work a long time further on and it is very expensive in your country.

FOR PATIENTS AND NEEDLES SAKE

Keep in your mind please, that each and every needle must be sterilized after use, if not you can cause severe infections with your next patient, Hepatitis or other ones. For sterilisation you have to use either a "Dry-Air-Sterilisator" for 1, 5 hours on 180 degrees Celsius . You can also put the needles in boiling water. The bubbles must be everytime coming up for one hour. The next way is a sterilisator working with vaporized water and compression for 20 minutes.

Keep your needles always tidy in a clean metal or glass box which you can close so that no dust can fall into in and the tips of the needles dont become bent.

FREQUENCY OF TREATMENT

Chronic diseases you should treat with Acupuncture once a weak. Acute diseases may be treated every second day. Of course you have to adjust to the constitution of the patient. Paralysis you can treat every day though it may exist since a long period.

One treatment should last for 20- 30 minutes. Thereafter the patient should better rest for another 15 - 30 minutes. If the patient has not reacted positively after the sixth treatment you have either chosen the wrong points or this disease can not be influenced by Acupuncture. This seldom is the case but it may be when the patient is taking cortison. At least you can always reduce pains even if you cannot cure the patient.

INDICATIONS AND CONTRAINDICATIONS

All diseases which are due to disturbance of the nerval or blood circulation can be helped. All pains, anaesthesia for operations, all diseases that could not be helped with other kinds of treatments in order to try everything possible.

Contraindicated are:
all diseases that can be better cured by other methods, such a tuberculosis, lepra or cancer. No treatment should be given in gravidity lest by an expert who knows the precautions in the special therapy for gravidity problems. If anatomical changes and destructions have taken place already, Acupuncture cannot cure them , such as arthrosis, rheumatism or others. But at least the pain can be reduced for some amount.

HINTS FOR THE RIGHT TECHNIQUE

The technique of how to insert the needles has to be learned with practical guidance. On dangerous aerias you have to insert the needles in a low angle. Where there is enough flesh, you can use an angle of 90 degrees.

The patient has to prepare himself for Acupuncture. The skin has to be kleen. If not, he first has to kleen it with water and perhaps with alkohol too. If you take the needles out again there may be some drops of blood coming out. Take a little clean piece of cotton and press for 2 minutes!

RECIPES

It has become clear that you must have complete diagnosis either by ayurvedic or chinese methods in order to decide which elements are missing in what point or channel or which elements are too much in which channel and this may differ in each patient. But there has been developed some kind of "Recipe -Acupuncture" for the beginner to make it easy for him. Those points are standard point combinations that may differ a lot for each patient but the chance that they help in this combination is quite good. I will tell you the most common diseases that you will deal with and the combination of points.

HINTS HOW TO USE THESE RECIPES

Try to use as few needles as possible. You do not necessarily have to use all the points mentioned. You can use them according to other symptoms as well, or to your experience or to the main pain location. In acute pains or diseases you can use more needles and at far-off places. In chronic diseases you should use less needles and in the neighbourhood of the affected part, as the body is already weakened.

Diarrhea	SP 4,ST 36, K6
Constipation	3F6, ST 25
Fever	DV 14, LI 4,11
Insomnia	DV 20, H7, BL 20
Sweating	H6, K7, LI 4
Nausea	CS 6, ST36
Hiccough	ST 36, CS 6, BL 17
Cervical pain (Channels SI+BL)	BL 10, DV 14, BL 11, SI 3,6,LU 7,LI 4,BL 60
(3F+ GB)	DV 14, GB 20, 21, 34, 39, 3F5, LI 4
Intercostal pain	LI 4, 3F8, GB 40, interrib-points (oblique)
Sciatica, lumbal pain (BL)	DV 3,4, BL 23, 26, 54, 36, 40, 60, 58, LI 4, Hand 1, 12
(GB)	DV 3,4, GB 30, 31, 34, 39, LI 4
Shoulder pain , frontal	DV 2, LI 4,,11, 14, 15, 16, ST 38
middle	3F 5,13, 14, LI 4, ST 38
dorsal	SI 3, 6, 9 DV ,14
Tennis elbow	LI 4, 11, LU 5, CS 3, H 3, 3F 5
Coxarthrosis	GB 30, 34, LI 4, BL 54, 32, 36, 40, 60, ST 44
Gonarthrosis	ST ,34, 35, 36 , 44, GB 34, BL 40, 11, 60, LI 4, Ex 31, 32
Rheumatoid Arthritis	3F 5, 15, LI 4

Respiratory Disorders (Asthma,Bronchitis)	LI 20, BL 2, LU 6, 7, LI 4, 3F5 , CV 17, 22, BL 17, ST 40, DV 14, H 7, CS 6
Common Cold	DV 14, 16, GB 20, LU 7, LI 4, 11, 3F 5, SP 10, Moxibustion: LI 11, CV 6, ST 36, K 7, BL 12
Sinusitis	LI 4, 11, 20, ST 2, 3, SI 18, SP 10, GB 14, BL 2, 60
Angina Pectoris	BL 15, CV 14, 17, CS 4, 6, H7
Hypertension	LIV 2, 3, 15, GB 20, LI 4, H7, ST 36
Hypotension	BL 23, CV 6, DV 11, 12, LI 10, 11, ST 36, K 7
Disturbance of Blood Supply in the Legs	GB 34, St 36, LU 9, 11, H 3, LI 4
Gastritis, Ulcer ventriculi	ST 34, 36, 21, 25, BL 21, LIV 13, 14, CS 6,
Mental disturbance	DV 20, H 7, CS 6, BL 15, 62, Ex 6
Agitation	Ex 6, BL 15, 62, H 5, 7, CS 6, LIV 3
Drug addiction	DV 14, 20, H 7, CS 6, LI 4, 3F 5, ST 36, GB 34, LIV 3 Ear-Point 55, 101, 100
Alkohol addiction	DV 20, CV 12, LIV 3, 13, 14, H 7, CS 6, ST 36, GB 34, Ear- Point 55, 84, 87, 98

Smoking addiction	DV 20, Ex 6, DV 14, H 7, CS 6
	Ear-Points 55, 87, 91, 101
Weakness symptoms, weight-loss	Moxibustion: BL 20, 21, 23, LIV 13, CV 12, GB 25, LI 11, St 36, K7
Headache (GB)	GB 14, 20, 41, 3F 5, LI 4
(ST)	ST 8, 36, 44, LI 4, 11
(BL)	BL 2, 10, 60, 67, SI 3, LI 4
Paralysis, Apoplexia	DV 20, Ex 6, LI 4, 11, ST 36, 38, BL 67, LIV 3, GB 34
	Skull-Acupuncture: along motoric zone/side of lesion
Epilepsy, acute attacks	DV 26
in intervals	DV20, 26, Ex 6,,1 H 7, CS 6, K61 ,GB 34, BL 62
Dysmenorrhea	CV 3, 4, 6, LI 4, SP 6, 10 , LIV 3, ST 36
Analgesia during Childbirth	DV 20, 2, 6, ST 29. CV 3, GB 21, LI 4, H 7, SP 6, LIV 3, ST 36, BL 67, Ex "Neima"
Skin Disorders	DV 14, SP 6, 10, LI 4, 11, LU 9
Fainting, Colapse	DV 26, CS 4, 9, H 9
Harmonizing of Hormones	BL 54, 60, LI 4, ST 36, SP 6, LIV 9, CS 5
Cramps	BL 2, 8, 10, GB 20, CV 15, DV 11, 19, 20, LIV 3

| Vertigo | CV 6, SI 5, ST 18, DV 19, GB 3, 20, BL 2, 10, 3F 23 |
| Toothache | LI 1, DV 26 |

ACUPUNCTURE IN THE VEDA AND AYURVEDA

More then 20 years ago when I first got in contact with Acupuncture, it was difficult for me to grasp the philosophical basics. Only when I became conversant with the Indian philosophy, the Vedanta and especially the Ayurveda I succeeded in this. Then I could suddenly understand that the medicals basics of both cultures are full of parallels and identical opinions. In the following pages the Sanskrit terms cannot explained in detail, so that the reader should consult one of the books from the list of literature.

History and Myth

As in the Chinese philosophy of Acupuncture we have the two founders Huang-Ti and Chi-Pai, we have a founder-pair of twins, the Ashvinas in Ayurveda, which mainly is derived as a medical science from the Rig-Veda and the Atharva-Veda. According to the standard textsbooks of Ayurveda Brahma explained this science to Prajapati Daksa in 100.000 verses and 1.000 chapters. The Ashwinas, the twin-godheads learnt it from him and taught it to Indra. Indra gave his knowledge to Rishi Bharadwaja who further handed it over to Atreya. Atreya had six disciples, one of them Agnisvesa, who let Caraka write the Caraka-Sangita (internal point of view of medicine). The two other classical texts are Susruta-Sangita (surgical point of view) and the Ashtangahridaya-Sangita (the only one translated into German language).

In a legend Susruta reports the following: Once the god of sacrifice, Yajna, wanted to perform a sacrifice for the welfare of heaven. He already had prepared everything in a wonderful manner, when out of a sudden Rudra, the god of war, grief and disease appeared und beheaeded Yajna. The other gods in heaven did not know what to do and so they asked the Ashvinas for help outside of heaven. They were twins and carpenters of the shoemakers caste. They sewed Yajnas head to the proper place again and out of gratefulness they got a heavenly abode as semi-godheads and thus became the first physicians.

The Ashvinas are mentioned several times in Rig-Veda. For example:

Ashvina no tri divyani bhesaja

(RV 1-34,6)

The medical translation of this vedic text (and for every science there is an individual key to unlock the Veda) means:

The Ashvinas can heal all the three kinds of ailments

Here the diseases which can affect the three doshas, Vata, Pitta and Kapha are referred to.

The foundation stone to both medical systems was thus laid by a pair of humans who cooperated in this. Huang-Ti and Chi-Pai on one side and on the other hand the Ashvinas.

The two divisions

An important subject in Acupuncture is the separation in the two opposites Yin and Yang. This dual aspect is existing in Ayurveda too. Here the uncreated God (Ram) when he wished to come into existence created two in opposite directions flowing rivers: Purusha and Prakriti, spirit and matter on which the whole creation is built up.

The three divisions

Chinese medicine knows three human types , who ca be affected by different diseases: The type of fullness, the type of emptiness and the balanced one. Acupuncture works with this concept in decreasing energy where there is too much, in increasing energy in channels where there is less and in balancing energy as a whole.

In this respect Ayurveda and Vedanta speak of Satvik, Tams and Rajas, referring to the physical aspect one talks of Vata, Pitta and Kapha. In the Veda these three aspects are also known . The knowing one (Rishi), the process of knowledge (Devata) and the object of knowledge (Chandas) have to be in balance, so that the unity of creation can prevail. So long as Vata, Pitta and Kapha are in balance, the man is healthy and the soul is able to understand the Veda (knowledge). Of course the Rig-Veda mentions these three factors quite often:

trayah paveyo madhuvahane rathe
somasya venamanu ita vishva viduh
trayah skambhitah skabhitasa
trinaktam stri ashvina diva yatha

(RV 1-34,2)

The medical translation means that we only can live in this
world with the three doshas. When they are in balance we can
gain health, if we act according to the medical advice
(Ashvinas). The three doshas are the three bodily aspects for all
human beings.

trih sobhagatvam trih uta shravansi

(RV 1-34,5)

The Veda says that the physicians keep the body in function by
balancing the three vital energys of Satva, Rajas and Tamas,
unimportant if the patient is of Kapha, Pitta or Vata constitution.

trih pathivanidattam adabhyam
omanam shamyo mamkaya sunave
tridhata sharma vahatam shubaspati

(RV 1-34,6)

And further it says: by such a medical advice we stay in such a
good health, that we are able to earn our own living and to fulfil
our wishes. Without being disturbed by pain we may
concentrate upon our own self.

Cosmic evolution and the concept of the five elements

The five elements are very common in the Veda and Ayurveda. Fire is identical with Agni, and earth with Prithvi, water with Jala or Aap. The fourth element is called Akash (Space, ether) and according to my understanding is identical with the element wood, as when a tree is growing, the energy of ether is working in order to built up a form and out of a non-space (the seed) produce a space consuming being (the tree). In the human body the wood-related organs liver and gall-bladder are are bulding up chemical forms too and thus are big factories in our body. the fifth element metal is identical with the vedic Vayu. This can be well understood from the metal-related organs lung and large intestine, which are in close contact with air.

It cannot be underestimated how exactly the Indian theory of evolution in addition to the Chinese circle of the five elements stands close to the scientific reality of today. Nowadays astronomy thinks that the universe out of its original form (Ram,Dao) split in matter and anti-matter(Ying/Yang, Purusha,Prakriti) with a great 'bang'. Thus the cosmos (Akasha) came into existence. Here balls of fire cristallized (Agni), out of which planets (Prithvi) were born. When these planets cooled down, mighty storms (Vayu) raised, which by differences in temperature in turn produced rains and oceans (Jala).

The human body is made of these five elements in deed which are not identical with chemical elements. 70 % of our body consists out of water (Jala), out of body-fluids. When it dies and is buried or burnt to ashes, it becomes earth (Prithvi) again. During life all processes of growth or production need the bodily warmth in the form of fire (Agni). Only by this the chemical factories in us can keep on working. The Jiva, the embodied soul cannot live for one moment without air (Vayu). Out of what the body is made else? A structure is necessary so that each organ knows, with what other organs it has to cooperate and in which way so that our body is getting and pertaining such a form which can be called 'human'. As science is teaching, more than 95 % off all matter is empty space in reality. Between electrons, atomic kernel and the neighbour atoms, out of which our body is made too, infinite distances exist as it is in the cosmic scale with solar systems and galaxies. This is the space-structure element (Ether/Akasha), which gives every created object its form.

Each of these elements is described in the Veda in so many verses.

pancha janah aditih vishvedeva
(RV 1-89,10)
indrah **pancha** kshitinam

(RV 1-7,9)

The meaning of the above is:

the creator resides in all the five planes of life.

Examples for the different elements in the Veda:

Earth:
> yesam ajmensu **prithvi** jujurvam iva
>
> (RV 1-37,8)

Wind or metal:
> esam janam **vayo** sthiram hi
>
> (RV 1-37,9)

Fire:
> **Agne** nah pitryani sakhya ma
>
> (RV 1-71,10)

Water:
> Gosu priyam **amritam** rakshamana
>
> (RV 1-71,9)

In the last verse "Amrit" is a synonym for "water", the "water of life". In Veda we find several other synonyms for the water element. "Soma" is another one. It is worthwile mentioning in this context that in the ancient European Greek language "soma" is standing for the human physical body, which needs the water of life.

Ether: the term "akasha" is found at several places of the Veda too.

In a German translation by Richter we find in RV 10-125 all the five elements together. Let me quote only the important passages:

> I carry Indra and **Agni** and the two Ashvins...
> I walk in **heavens** (Akasha) and the **earth**...
> My lap is in the **water**, inmidst of the ocean...
> I blow as the **wind**.

And in RV 10-85:

Vayu is the protector of **soma** (water)...
Heaven (Akasha) and **earth** were her chariot,
when the sun´s daughter (embodied soul) travelled to her
groom...
and **Agni** was her leader

The 107 Marmas of Ayurveda and Acupuncture

As the channels in Chinese Acupuncture Ayurveda knows the existence of Srotas and Nadis, which are not always visible for human eyes, as it is with the Chinese channels. The two important Acupuncture channels Conception and Director Vessel respond to the Sanskrit terms Ida and Pingala, as can be understood by the postulated functions of the same. Indian medicine knows 107 important "Marmas", the location of which is exactly described in the classics of Ayurveda and is always identical with the location of an important Acupuncture point. They respond to Acupuncture points also because of the fact that their injury has the same effects - as described by Susruta- as the indication for the usage of the Acupuncture points situated at the same place. For example: A Marma which when enjured led to a paretic leg can as an Acupuncture point be used for treatment of paresis in legs. It seems to be a similar mechanism as in Homoeopathy; the dosage makes the poison. But why Susruta only describes the results of injuries? This can be explained when knowing, that Susruta had mainly to care for injured soldiers as a war surgeon. The healing effect of treatment at the Marmas was known still. Massage of these places and cauterisation was described and are still in use today. In India I met a 80-year old patient, who suffered from epilepsy in childhood. A village-healer cured this disease out of a sudden by burning a small hole in his ear .(Ear Acupuncture was newly discovered by the French doctor Nogier). Another patient had a sciatica in childhood which went away within a second by cauterisation of another ear-point. This place was identical to a nowadays well-known point for the lumbar spine.

Though in Chinese Acupuncture much more Acupuncture points are investigated and described, the ancient Ayurveda talks only of 107 Marmas, which are the most important ones. Where do we find this 107 mentioned in the Veda?

In the German poet Rückert's translation of the Atharva-Veda 4-16 it is said:

> Varuna, your **seven** snares are triple set for hunting,
> to entangle the untruthful.
> The truthful shall be freed.
> With **hundred** snares cath the wicket, Varuna!

Seven snares plus 100 snares are 107 Marmas by which the wicket diseases can be cured. They are triple set because of the three doshas which must be taken into account as everyone is of another constitution. They are triple set also because of the methods of tonification, sedation and balancing known in Acupuncture.

The same author translated Atharva-Veda 13-2:

> Hail thee, oh sun, when you drive over the skies.
> Your chariot is moved by **107** horses.
> The very best ones were chosen.

Though Rückert´s translation sometimes is so chaotic, that it really seems to become a book of witch craft as it is believed to be by the western scholars, we can understand what is meant in medical terms.

The human body is praised as a chariot, driven by the embodied soul. The most important 107 points of Acupuncture or the Marmas are mentioned, by which the body can be influenced in order to stay healthy throughout the time of the stay on this planet earth.

All the 107 Marmas and their linking channels are later being described in the classical ayurvedic texts. See Vagbhatas Astangahridaya- Sangita Sarirasthana,4 th chapter, Caraka-Sangita , Vimanasthana, 5 th chapter and Susruta-Sangita, Salya-Tantra, Marmasthana. According to Susruta there are five types of Marmas which when afflicted lead to the following defects:

1. Sadhyapranahara (immediate loss of conciousness, death within one day)
2. Kalantara (slowly progression of death)
3. Vaikalyakara (changing life giving processes to bad)
4. Visalyagna (something coming from outside has to be integrated by time into the body forming scars)
5. Rujakara (by injury pain is resulting)

Further parallels

As well as in the Chinese as in the ayurvedic texts one finds a cycle of the body functions and the engery flow during the time. This fact has to be kept in mind when influencing different diseases so that the balance of the five elements is regained.

Pulse-diagnose is not only propagated by Chinese doctors, but is described in the ayurvedic texts in a modified manner with an exact mentioning of the various pulse qualities in so many diseases.

Conclusion

All kinds of science where existing since the beginning of the world in a hidden cryptic form as it is with the seed of a fruit. According to the development and needs of the age (yuga) wise men can water the seed and bring it to maturity. The semen wears in its kernel already the whole (The Microcosm is in the Macrocosm). When in former periods of history India and China were one big cultural unit, the teaching of the five elements was developed out of the knowledge of the Veda, and with it the Ayurveda as the medicine for the people. The Marma-therapy namely Acupuncture is a special technique of the former. Acupuncture and the medical philosphy on which it is based, is not purely of Chinese origin. The texts of Veda which are dated still further back than the first Chinese ones as well as the contemporary Ayurvedic texts (2000 b.C.) give many hints that these thought were moved already much earlier. Thus it can be assumed that Acupuncture was practised already 5.000 or 10.000 years ago ,long before the Mahabharata war which had destroyed a worldwide culture of high standards in a cultural context that comprised at least both the regions of India and China today.

APPENDIX

THE FIRST INSTRUMENTS OF THE STARTING ACUPUNCTURER

50 stainless steel needles

Clean cotton

A Cunmetre

An instrument for electric point detection

A metal or otherwise good closing and clean box for the needles

Desinfection fluid or pure alkohol

This book, to look up what you cannot keep in mind

LOCALISATION OF THE MOST IMPORTANT POINTS

Here I will list the most important points of each channel and the location measured in Cun. Some anatomical knowledge with the medical terms in Latin may be needed.

LUNG CHANNEL

LU 1	6 Cun lateral to the midline and in relaxed shoulder 1 Cun below the clavicle and 1 Cun below LU 2
LU 5	At the elbow crease lateral to the biceps tendon
LU 6	7 Cun proximal to the wrist crease on the radial side of the forearm
LU 7	On radial side of forearm at the border of the radius,1,5 Cun proximal to the transverse crease of the wrist
LU 11	Just at the radial side nail corner of the thumb (2 mm)

LARGE INTESTINE CHANNEL

LI 1	At the radial nail corner of the second finger (2mm)
LI 2	On the radial side of the base joint of the second finger in a small pitch (let patient make a fist)
LI 4	At the highest point of muscle adductor pollicis with thumb and 2 nd Finger abducted
LI 6	3 Cun proximal ton the backside of the forearm and proximal of the opposite side of wrist-crease
LI 7	2 Cun proximal to LI 6
LI 11	On the transverse crease between the middle of biceps tendon and the lateral condyle of humerus (forearm flexed to a right angle
LI 15	With the arm abducted in the shoulder in the anterior depression
LI 18	3 Cun lateral to the prominence of the thyroid cartilage
LI 19	Below the nose 0, 5 Cun lateral to DV 26
LI 20	Between ala nasi and nasal labial groove

STOMACH CHANNEL

ST 2	on the infraorbital foramen
ST 3	Directly below ST 2 at the lower border of the ala nasi
ST 4	0, 5 Cun lateral to the corner of the mouth on the vertical line below the middle of the eyebrow
ST 5	At the lowest point of the anterior border of the Masseter Muscle
ST 6	At the midpoint of the Masseter Muscle when the jaw is closed
ST 8	0, 5 Cun close to the hairlineedge on forehead, 4, 5 Cun lateral of the midline and 3 Cun above eyebrows
ST 21	2 Cun lateral to the midline, 4 Cun above the navel
ST 25	2 Cun lateral to the navel
ST 29	4 Cun directly below ST 25
ST 35	In the depression lateral to the lower patella-border when the knee is slightly bent
ST 36	0, 5 Cun lateral to the tuberositas tibiae, 3 Cun below the knee-joint
ST 38	5 Cun below ST 36, 0,5 Cun lateral to the anterior border of the tibia
ST 40	0,5 Cun lateral to ST 38, 2 Cun lateral to the tibial border, 5 Cun below ST 36
ST 44	0,5 Cun proximal of the margin of the web between the 2 nd and 3 rd metatarsal bone
ST 45	On the lateral corner of the border of 2 nd toenail

SPLEEN CHANNEL

SP 1	On the inner side of the big toe on the nail corner
SP 2	On the inner side on the big toe on the borderline between red and white flesh, at the end of base bone
SP 3	Proximal to the head of the 1 st metatarsal bone on the medial side of the foot
SP 4	In the depression distal to the base of 1 st meta-tarsal bone on the medial side of the foot
SP 6	3 Cun above the medial ankle, dorsal to the posterior border of the tibia
SP 8	3 Cun below SP 9
SP 9	Medial side of leg in depression below the lower border of the medial condyle at the level of tube-rositas tibiae
SP 10	The highest point of the muscle vastus medialis, 2 Cun proximal of the upper patella border
SP 15	4 Cun lateral to the navel,lateral to ST 25

HEART CHANNEL

H 5	1 Cun proximal to H7, radial to the tendon of muscle carpi ulnaris
H 6	0,5 proximal to H 7
H 7	On the transverse to the wrist, radial to the tendon of muscle carpi ulnaris,needling is also possible from the ulnar side of the wrist, lateral to the tendon of mscle carpi ulnaris
H 9	radial side of the nail-corner of the middle finger

SMALL INTESTINE CHANNEL

SI 1	At the outer nail corner of the small finger
SI 3	On the ulnar border of the hand with the fist clenched at the ulnar end of the main transverse crease of palm
	This point is located proximal to the head of the os metacarpale toward the ulna
SI 4	On the ulnar side of the back of the hand between the basic joint of 5 th finger and os hamatum in a small ditch
SI 6	In the depression of the radial side of the styloid process
SI 7	5 Cun proximal of the transverse of the wrist on the backside of the hand just between SI 5 and SI 8
SI 8	On the back of the elbow joint in a ditch between olecranon and the tip of the medial epicondyle (elbow bent)
SI 9	When the arm is abducted 1 Cun above the dorsal crease of the axilla
SI 18	Distal to the arcus zygomaticus ,directly below the outer canthus of the eye

BLADDER CHANNEL

BL 2	On the medial end of the eyebrow directly above the inner corner of the eye
BL 10	1, 75 Cun lateral to DV 15
BL 13	1,5 Cun lateral to the lower border of the spinous process of T III
BL 14	1,5 Cun lateral to the lower border of the spinous process of T IV
BL 15	1,5 Cun lateral to the lower border of the spinous process of T V
BL 16	1,5 Cun lateral to the lower border of the spinous process of T VI
BL 17	1,5 Cun lateral to the lower border of the spinous process of T VII
BL 18	1,5 Cun lateral to the lower border of the spinous process of T IX
BL 19	1,5 Cun lateral to the lower border of the spinous process of T X
BL 20	1,5 Cun lateral to the lower border of the spinous process of T XI
BL 21	1,5 Cun lateral to the lower border of the spinous process of T XII
BL 23	1,5 Cun lateral to the lower border of the spinous process of L II
BL 22	1,5 Cun lateral to the lower border of the spinous process of L I
BL 25	1,5 Cun lateral to the lower border of the spinous process of L IV
BL 27	1,5 Cun lateral to the posterior midline at the level of the S I sacral foramen

BL 28	1,5 Cun lateral to the posterior midline at the level of the S II sacral foramen
BL 40	At the middle of the popliteal transverse crease on the back of the knee
BL 58	Just 7 Cun above BL 60
BL 60	At the middle of the connecting line drawn between the outer ankle and the achilles tendon
BL 62	0, 5 Cun directly below the outer ankle
BL 67	At the lateral nail corner of the little toe

KIDNEY CHANNEL

K 1	On the sole of the foot between the middle and last third of the sole
K 3	Midway between the most prominent point muscle soleus medialis and the superior border of achilles tendon
K 4	10 mm under and behind K 3
K 5	1 Cun just below K 3
K 6	1 Cun directly below the tip of the inner ankle
K 7	On the anterior border of achilles tendon and 2 Cun above the inner ankle

THE CHANNEL OF CIRCULATION/SEXUALITY

CS 1   1 Cun lateral of the nipple in the fourth interco-
            stal space
CS 4   Between the tendons of the muscles palmaris
            longus and muscle flexor carpi radialis, 5 Cun
            proximal of the transverse crease of the wrist
CS 6   Between the tendons of muscle palmaris longus
            and flexor carpi radialis ,2 Cun proximal to the
            transverse crease of the wrist
CS 7   On the transverse crease of the wrist between the
            tendons of m.palmaris longus and m.flexor carpi
            radialis.
CS 9   On the radial nail corner of the middle finger

THE CHANNEL OF THREE FIRES

3 F 1   On the inner nail corner of the ring finger
3 F 3   On the back of the hand between the 4th and 5th
            metacarpal bones proximal to the metacarpopha-
            langeal joint.
3 F 4   1/2 Cun proximal to 3F 3
3 F 5   On the midpoint between ulna and radius, 2 Cun
            proximal to the dorsal crease of the wrist
3 F 6   Between ulna and radius, 3 Cun proximal to the
            wrist
3 F 7   1 finger width lateral to 3 F 6 on the radial
            border of the ulna
3 F 8   Between ulna and radius, 4 Cun proximal of the
            wrist

3F 10	1 Cun behind and over the olecranon in a ditch, with the elbow bent
3F 14	The more dorsal situated of the two depressions palpable to the shoulder when the arm is abducted.
3F 15	On the middle line between the tip of the acromion to DV 14, 1 Cun below GB 21.
3F 17	In the depression posterior to the ear lobe, anterior to the mastoid process
3F 21	When the mouth is opened in the depression anterior to the intertragic nodge, above the condyle process of the mandibula

GALLBLADDER CHANNEL

GB 1	1/2 Cun lateral to the outer corner of the eye
GB 2	When the mouth is opened the point is palpable in a depression behind the mandibula
GB 14	On the forehead 1 Cun above the midpoint of the eyebrow
GB 20	Between the origins of M.sternocleidomastoideus and M.trapezius
GB 21	At the highest point of the shoulder between the prominence (DV 14) and the acromion
GB 23	Infront of GB 22 in the 4 th intercostal space
GB 24	On the mamillary line ,7 th intercostal space
GB 25	On the lower border of the free end of the 12 th rib
GB 26	Midway between the free ends of the 11 th and the 12 th rib, at the level of the navel
GB 30	On the line from the major trochanter to the lower border of the sacral bone, at the border between the outer and middle thirds of this distance
GB 34	On the point of intersection of the lines of the anterior and inferior borders of the fibular head.
GB 36	1 Cun behind GB 34 at the back border of the fibula on the midway between GB 34 and the outer ankle
GB 37	On the anterior side of the fibula, 5 Cun proximal of the outer ankle
GB 38	4 Cun above the outer ankle, on the frontal border of the fibula

GB 39	Between the posterior border of the fibula and the tendons of m.peroneus longus and m. peroneus brevis, 3 Cun proximal of the outer ankle
GB 40	3 mm infront and below the outer ankle in a ditch, lateral to the tendon of m.extensor digitorum longus
GB 41	Distal to the base and between the 4 th and 5 th metatarsal bones
GB 43	Between the 4th and 5 th toe, 10 mm behind the web of the both toes
GB 44	2 mm on the outer nail-corner of the 4th toe

LIVER CHANNEL

LIV 1	On the lateral side of the big toe on its midth
LIV 2	Between 1 st and 2 nd toe, 10 mm proximal of the the web
LIV 3	Between the 1 st and 2 nd metatarsal bones, 2 Cun proximal of the margin of the web
LIV 6	7 Cun over the tip of the inner ankle on the backside of the tibia
LIV 8	On the inner end of the transverse popliteal crease at the anterior border of m.semimembranosus and m.semitendinosus
LIV 9	4 Cun over the inner femoral condyle between m. sartorius and m.vastus medialis
LIV 13	At the free end of the 11 th rib
LIV 14	On the mamillary line in the 6 th intercostal space

DIRECTOR VESSEL

DV 4	Between the spinous process of L2 and L3
DV 6	Below the spinous process of T11
DV 11	Below the spinous process of T5
DV 13	Below the spinous process of t 1
DV 14	Below the spinous process of C7 (vertebra pro-minens)
DV 20	On the continuation of the line connecting the highest points of the ears, on the head's midline, 7 Cun above the posterior hairline, 5 Cun behind the anterior hairline
DV 26	At the border of the middle and upper thirds of the distance between the nose and the upper lip

CONCEPTION VESSEL

CV 3	On the midline, 1 Cun above the symphysis
CV 4	On the midline 3 Cun below the navel
CV 6	On the midline, 1,5 Cun below the navel
CV 8	Directly on the navel (forbidden point, only used for moxibustion)
CV 12	On the midline between the xyphoid process and the navel, 4 Cun above the navel
CV 14	On the midline, 6 Cun above the navel
CV 17	On the middle of the breastbone, between the nipples, on the level of the 4 th intercostal space
CV 22	In the fossa jugularis
CV 23	Midway between the upper border of the cricoid cartilage and the lower border of the mandibula

EXTRA POINTS

Extra 1	Between the eyebrows on the midline at the root of the nose
Extra 6	4 points, located 1 Cun anterior,posterior, lateral to DV 20
Extra 8	for insomnia; between 3F 17 and Extra 7, 0,5 Cun dorsal to 3 F 17
Hand 1	2 points, each 1,5 Cun distal to the dorsal crease of the wrist ,between 1st and 2nd and 3rd and 4 th os metacarpale respectively
Hand 12	On the dorsal side of the hand between 4th and 5th head of ossa metacarpalia, a little bit closer to the 4 th . Hand 1 and 12 serve especially against sciatic pain

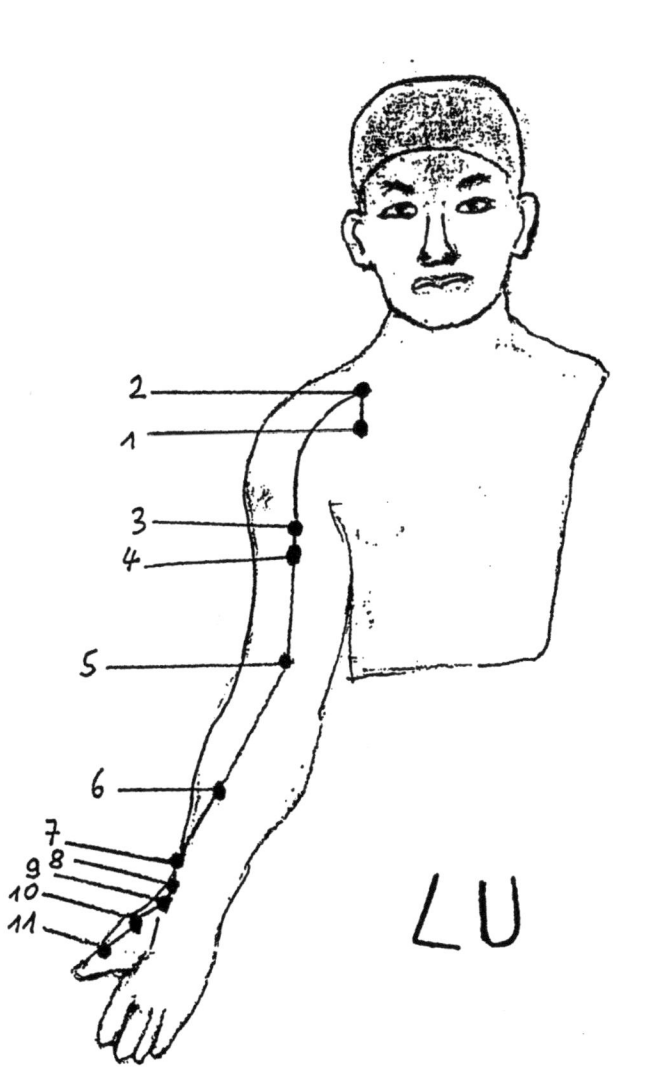

LU

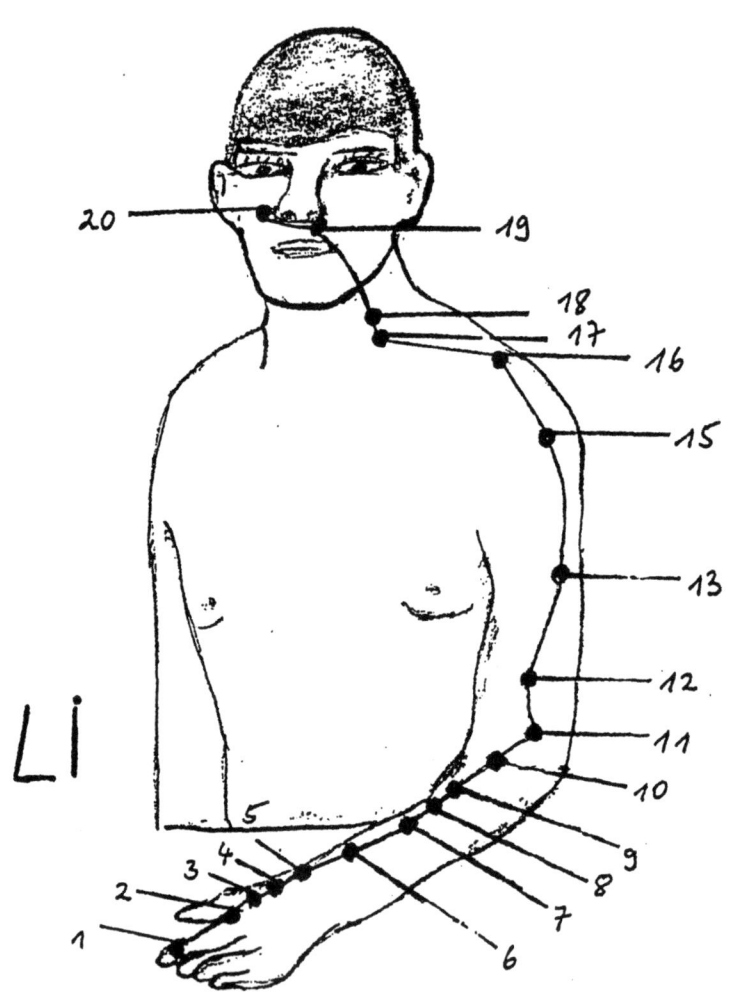

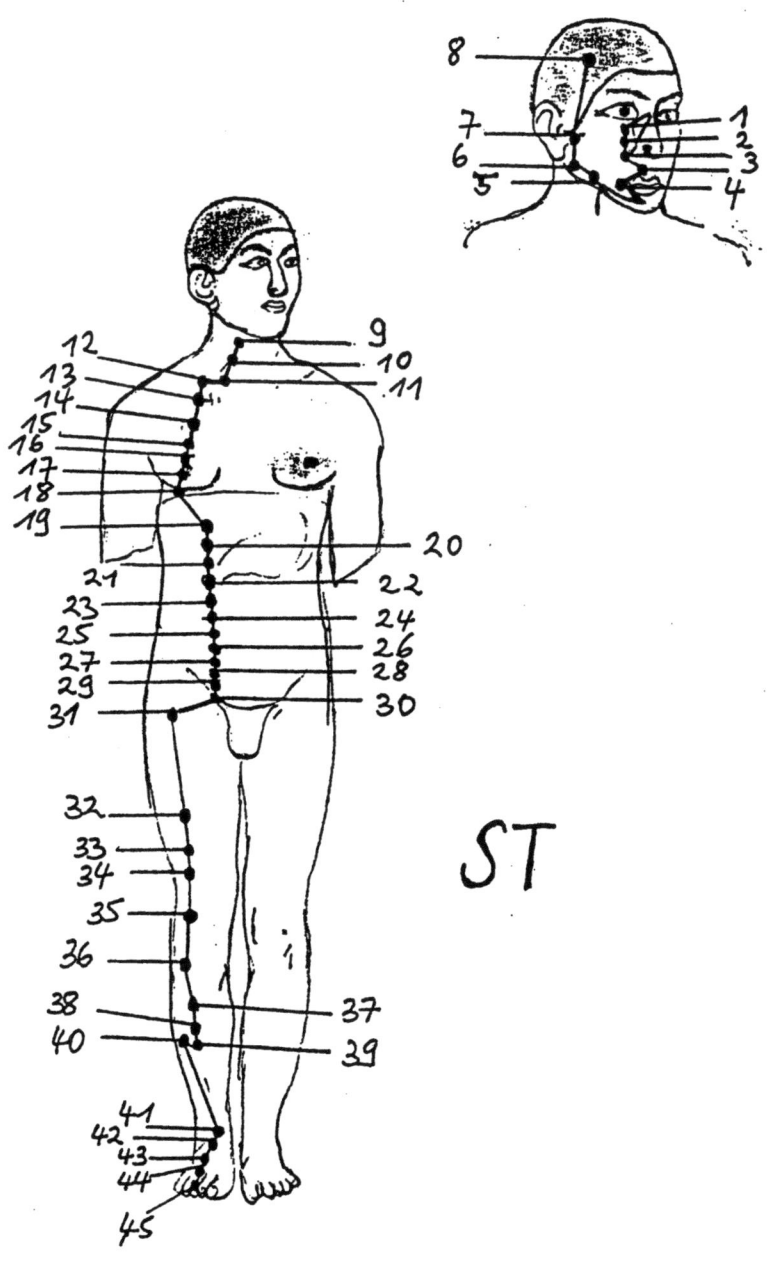

ST

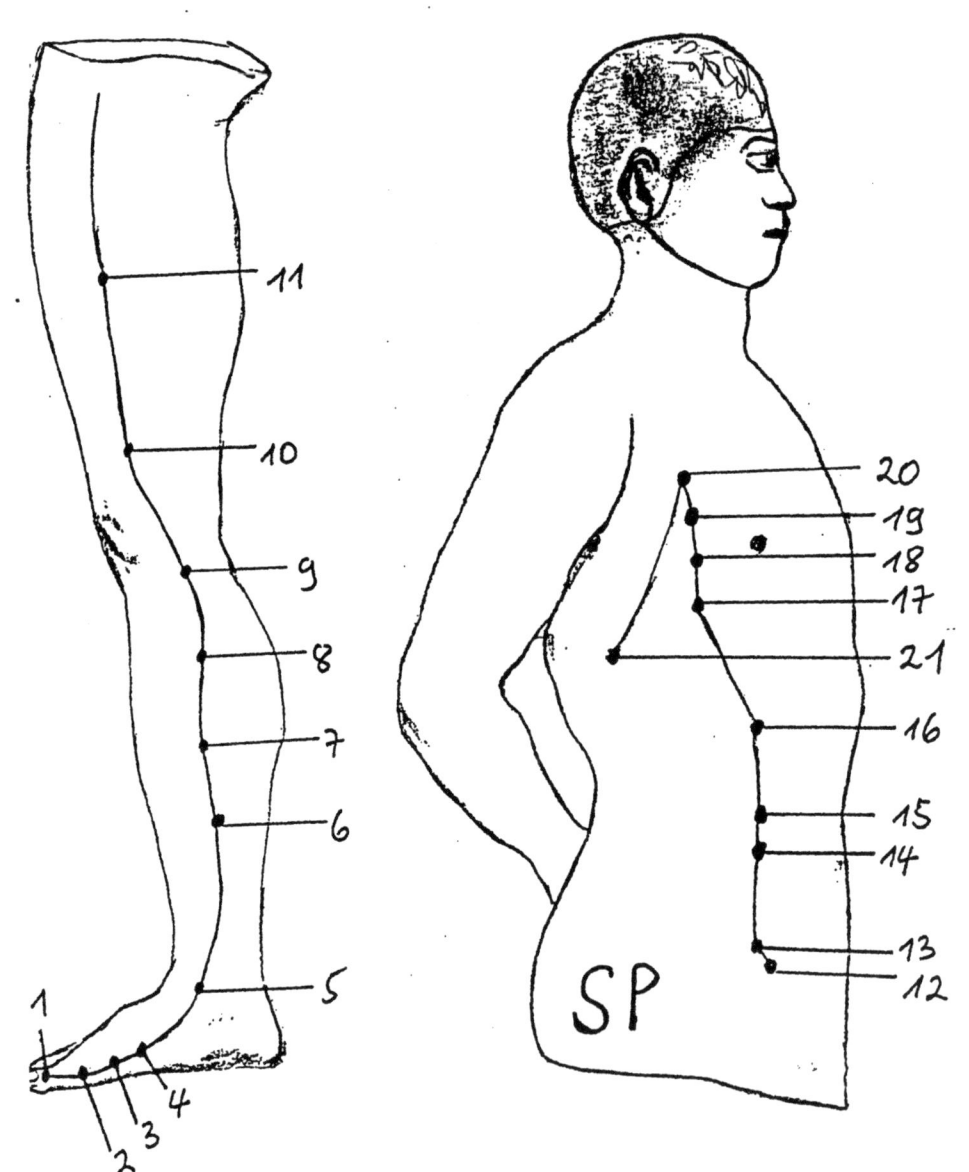

SP

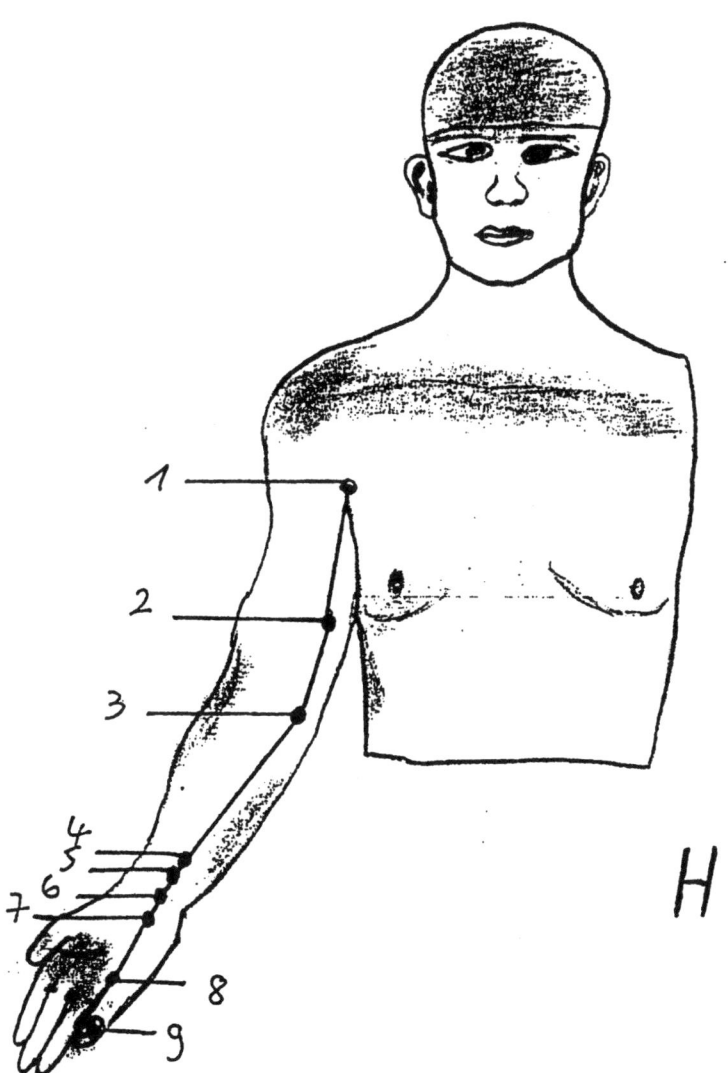

H

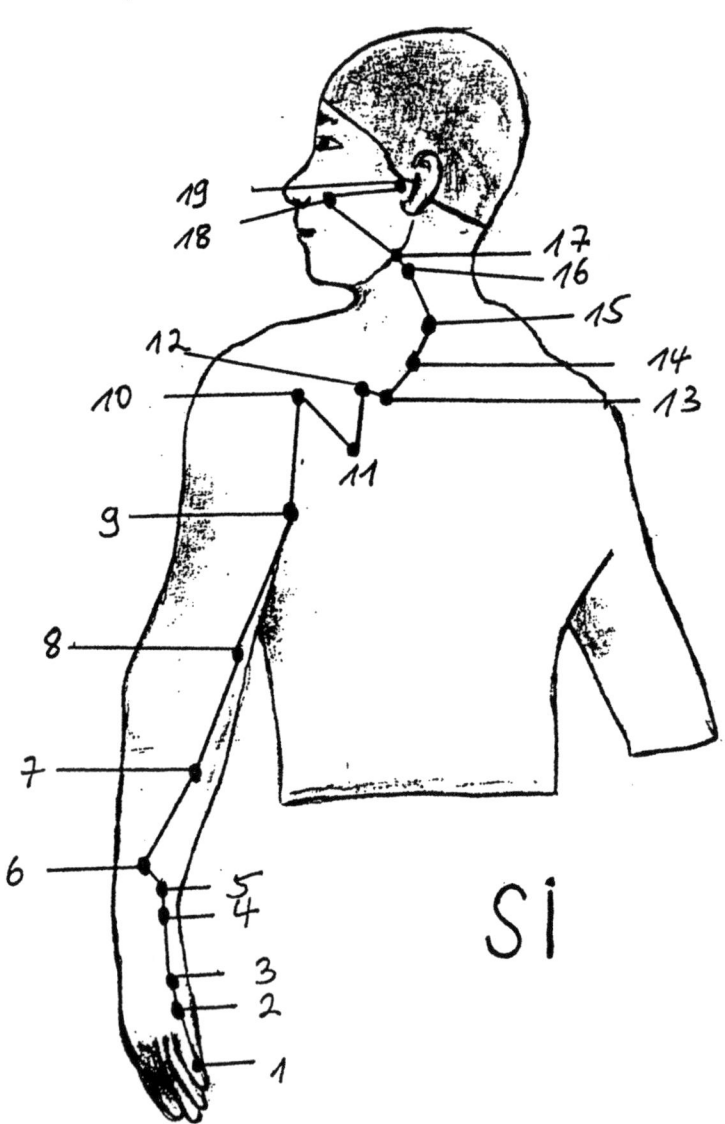

Si

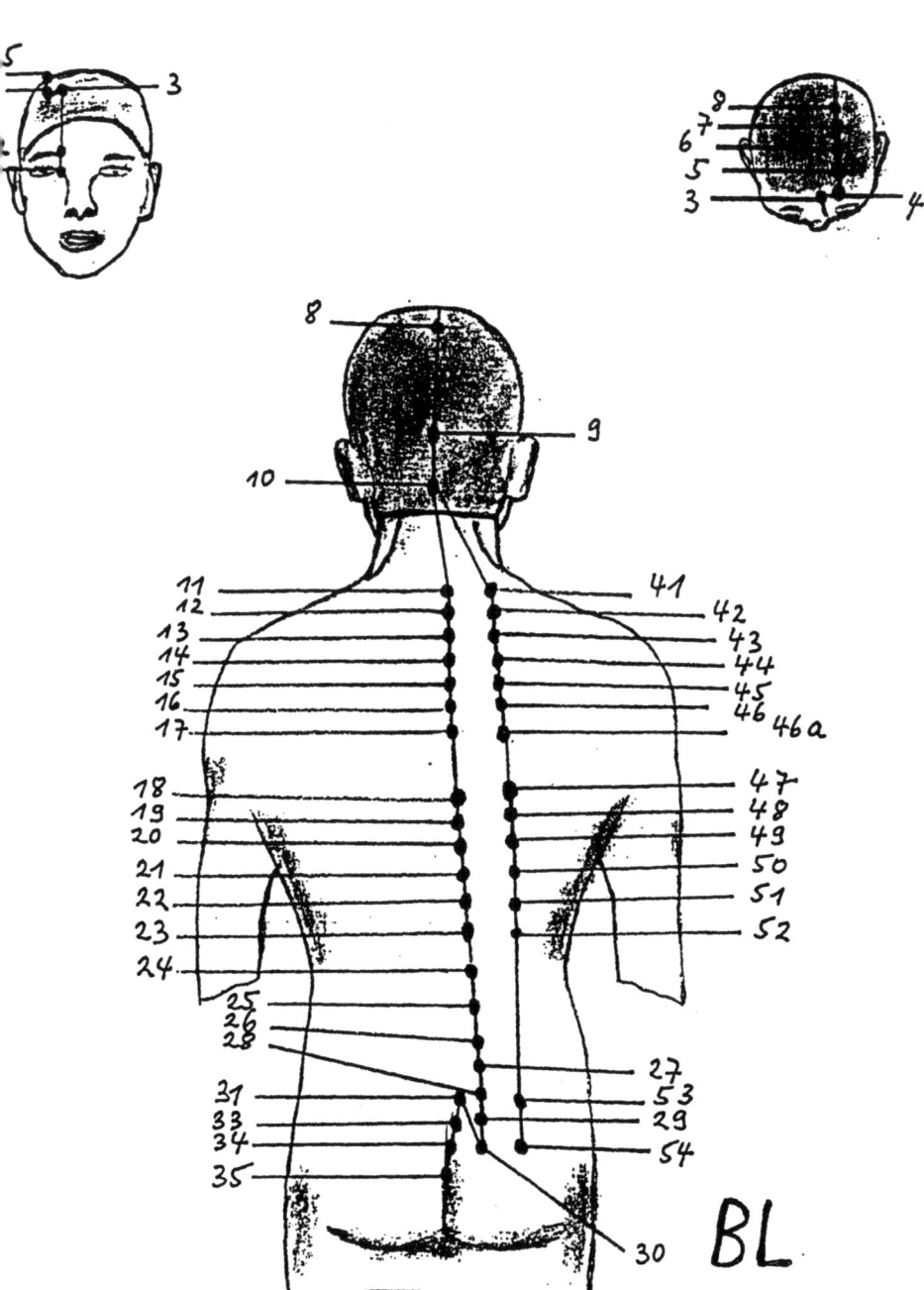

BL

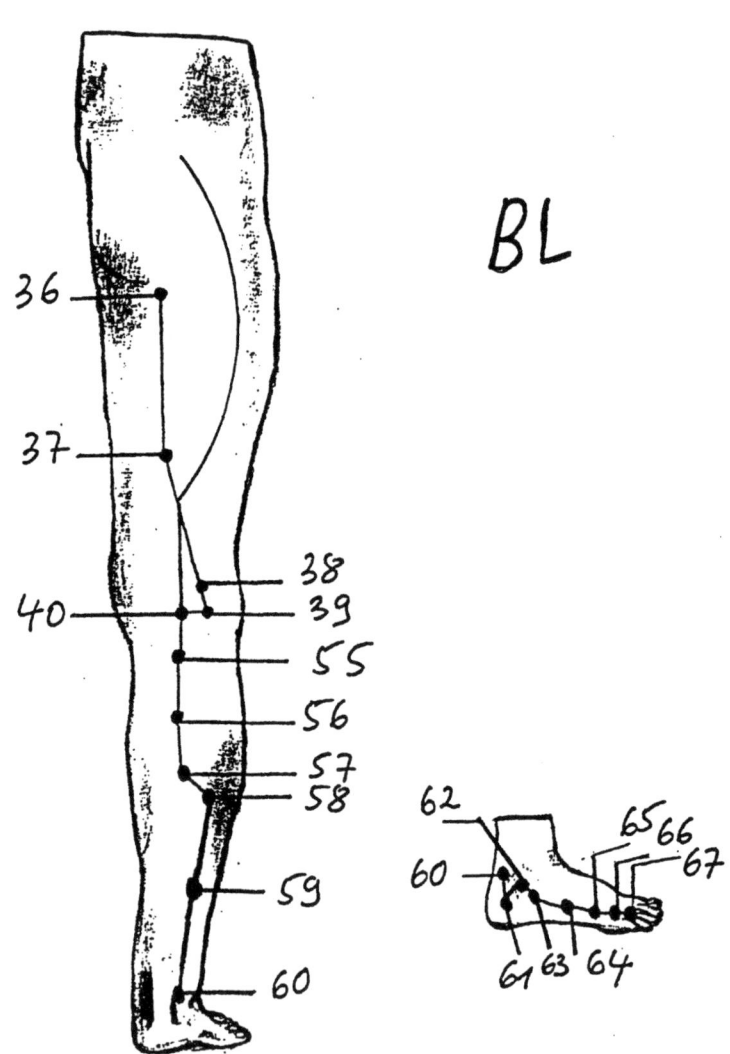

BL

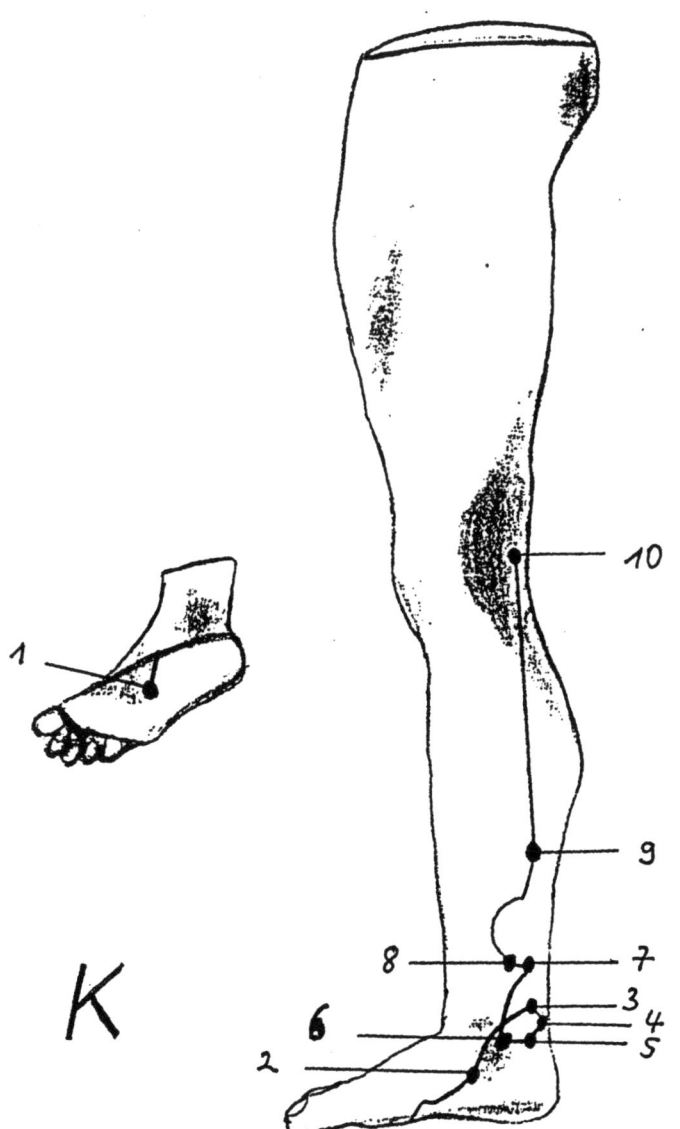

K

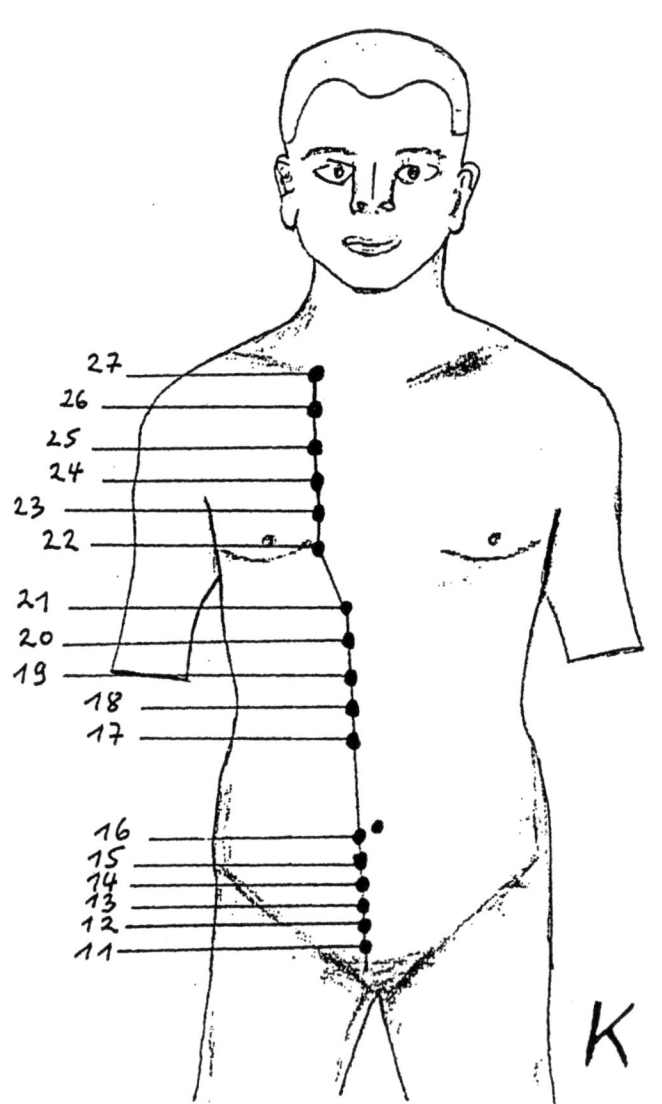

27 ——————
26 ——————
25 ——————
24 ——————
23 ——————
22 ——————

21 ——————
20 ——————
19 ——————

18 ——————
17 ——————

16 ——————
15 ——————
14 ——————
13 ——————
12 ——————
11 ——————

K

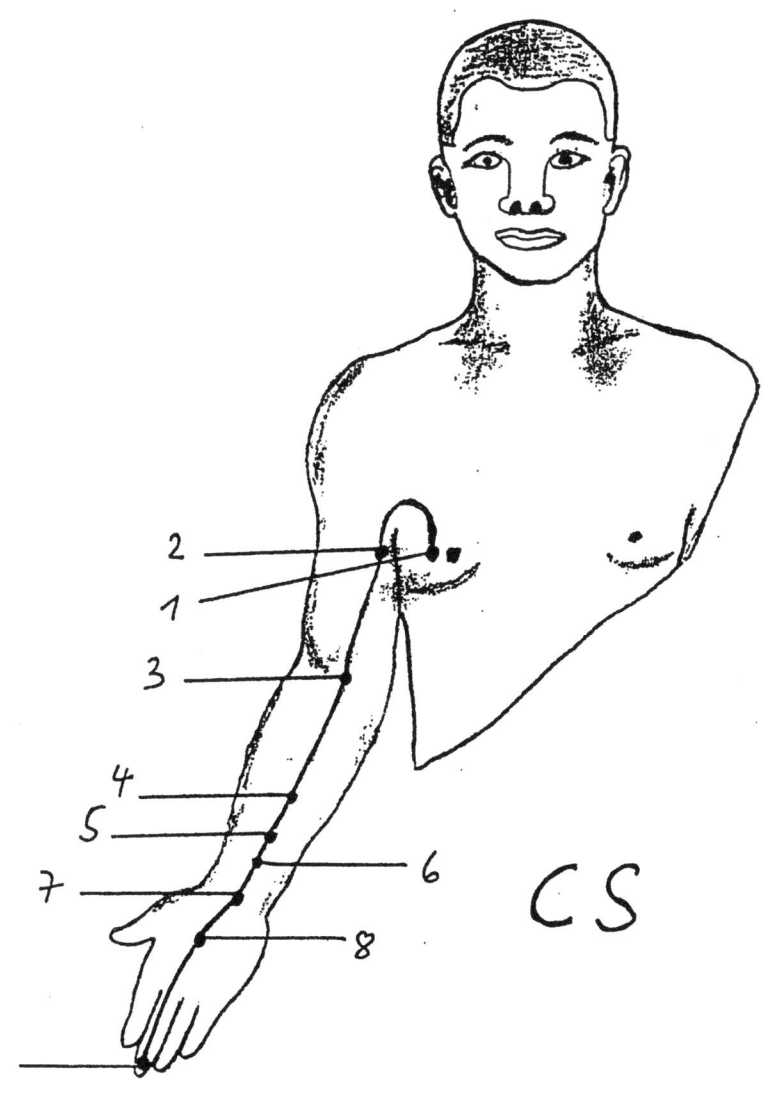

CS

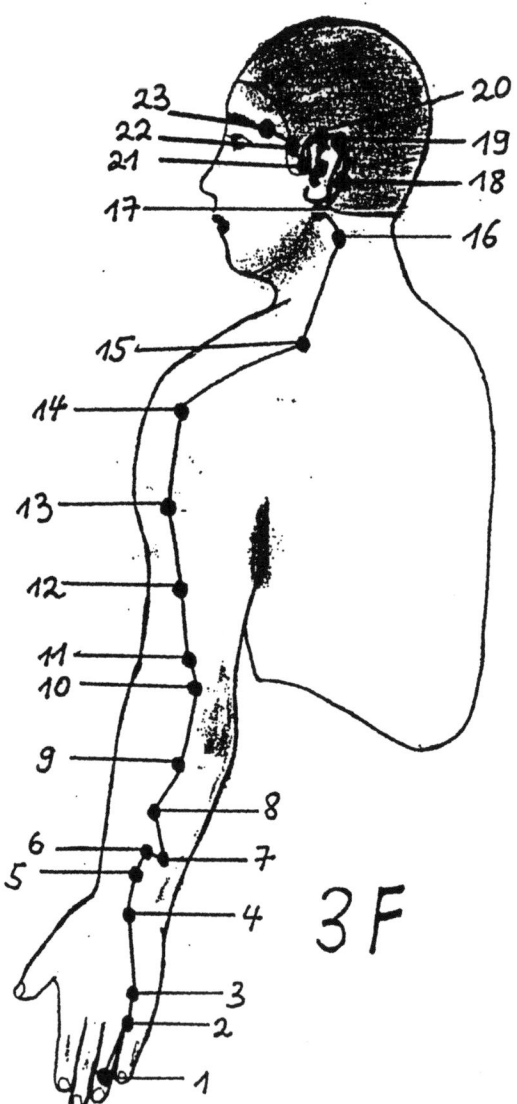

3F

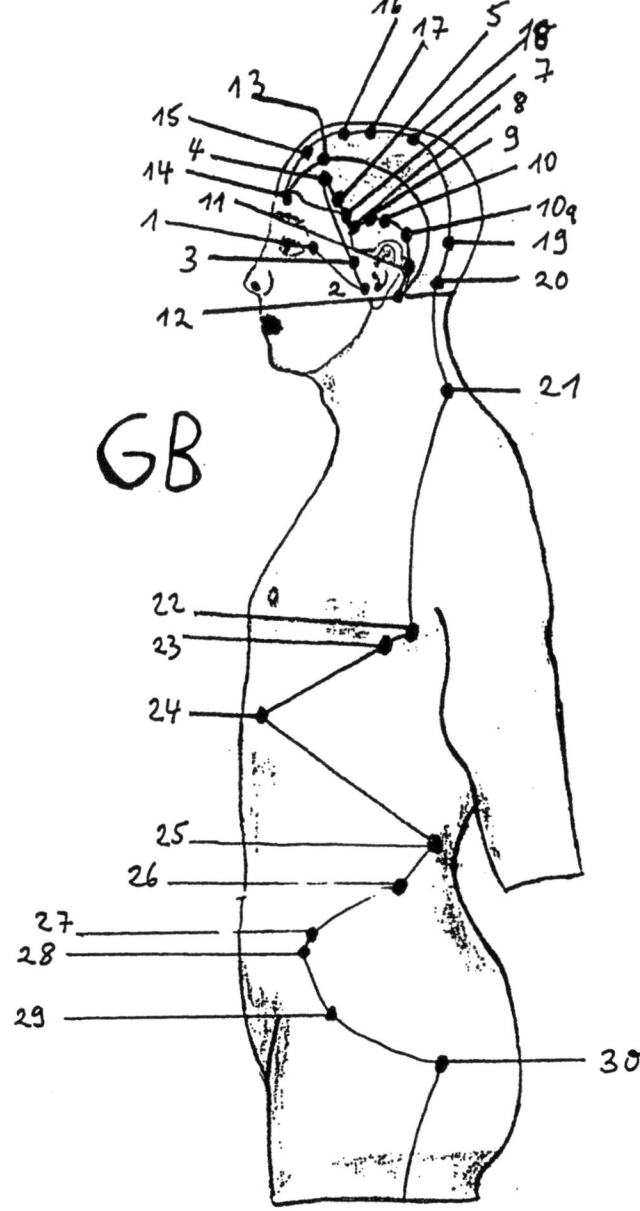

GB

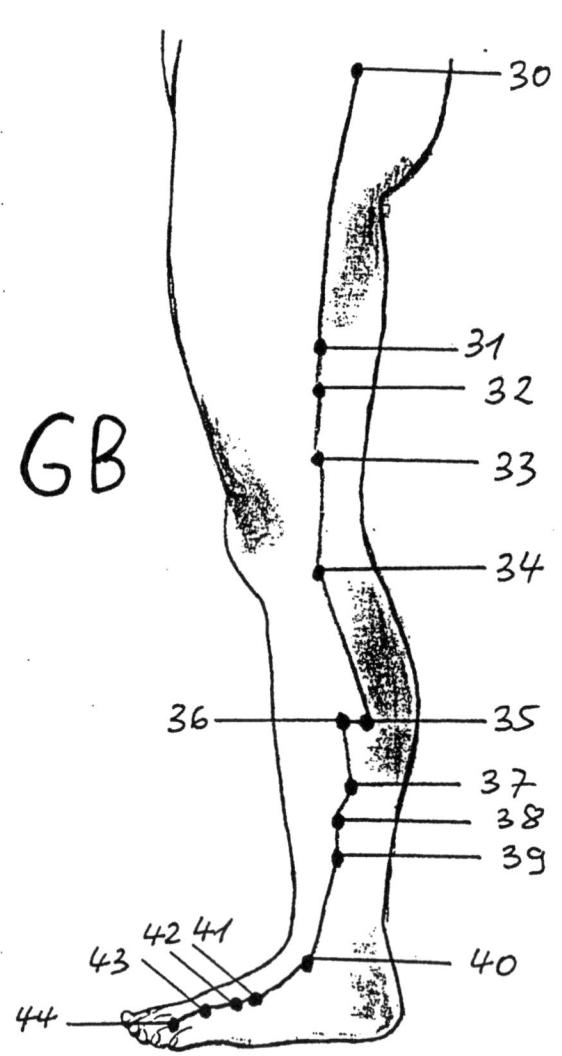

GB

30

31
32
33
34
36 — 35
37
38
39
42 41
43 40
44

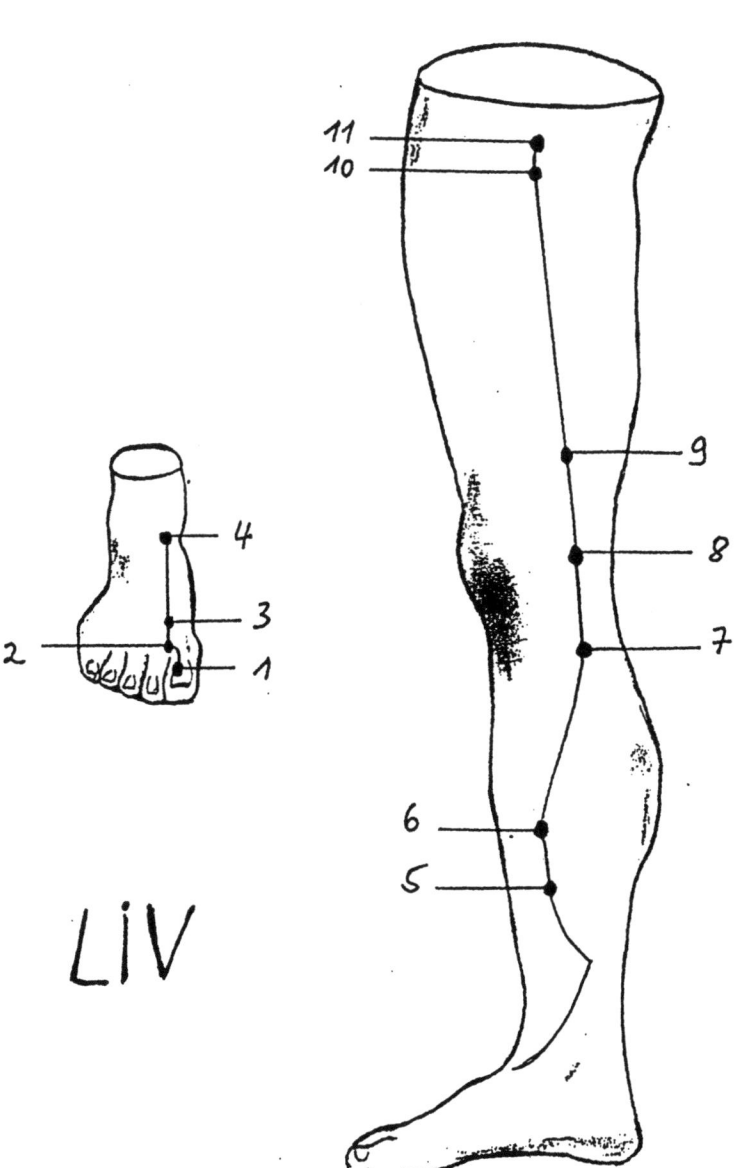

LiV

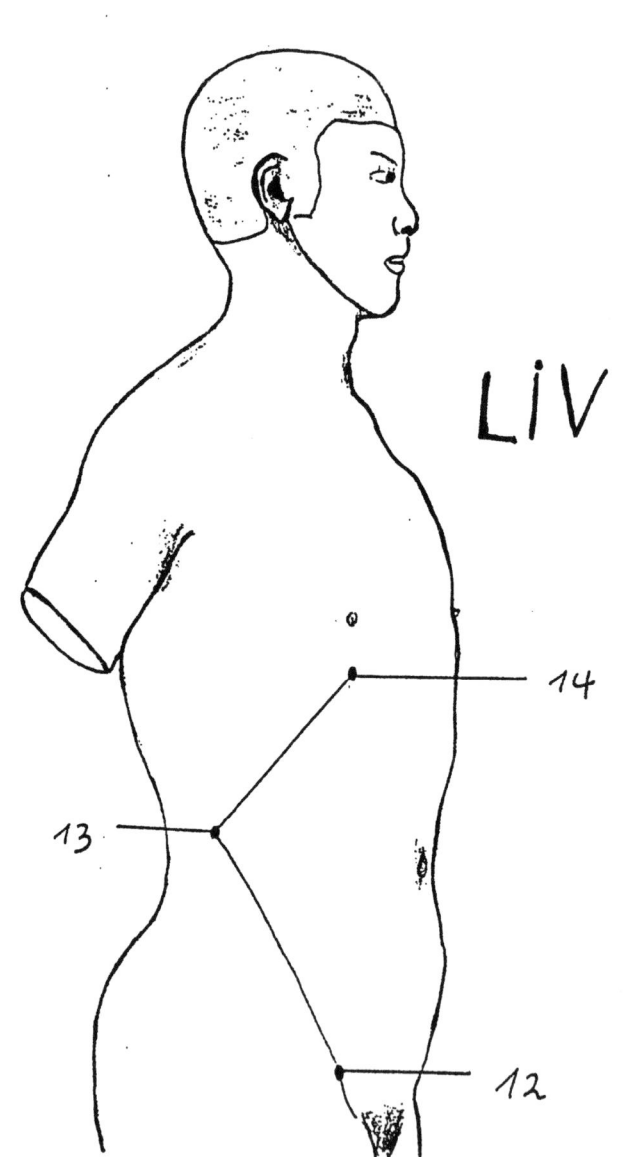

LIV

14

13

12

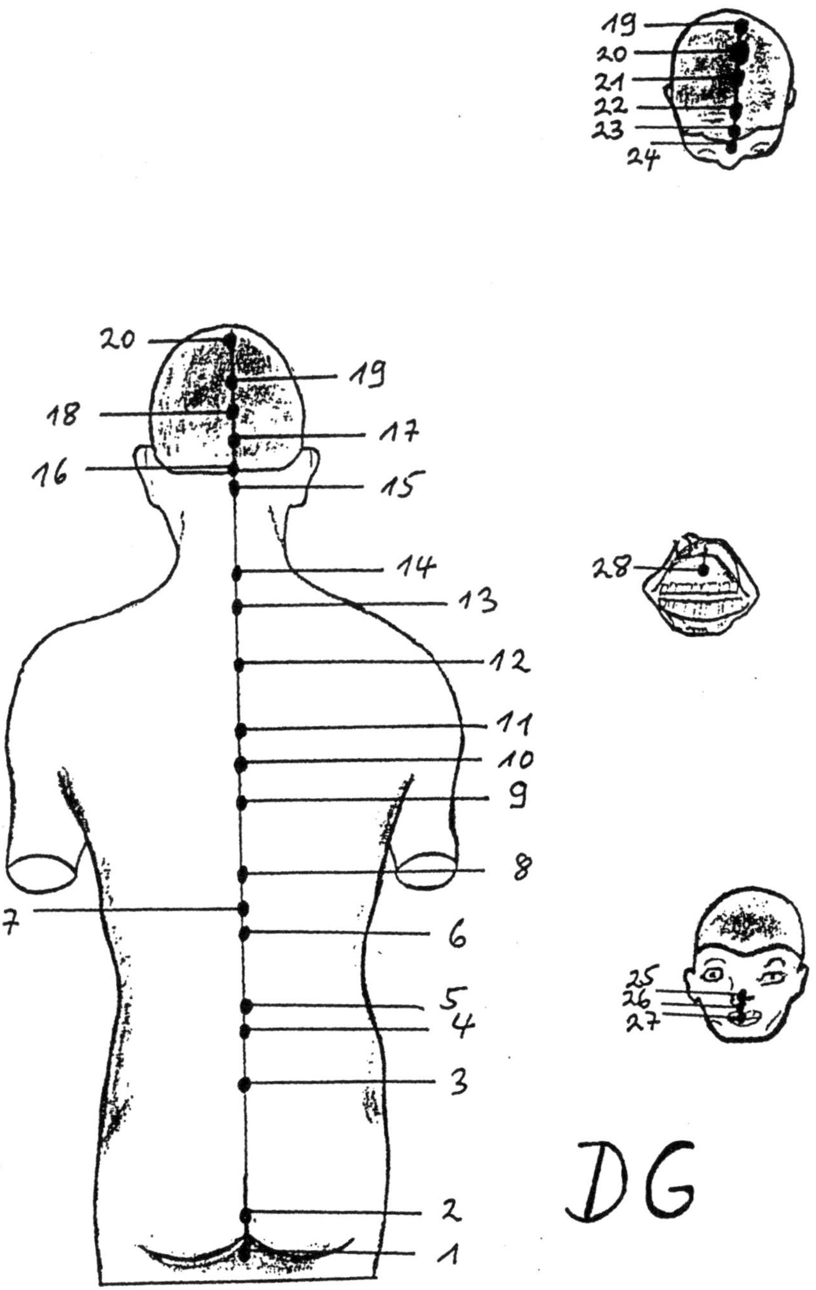

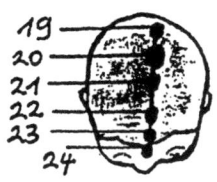

19
20
21
22
23
24

20

18

16

19

17

15

14

13

12

11

10

9

8

6

5
4

3

2

1

7

28

25
26
27

DG

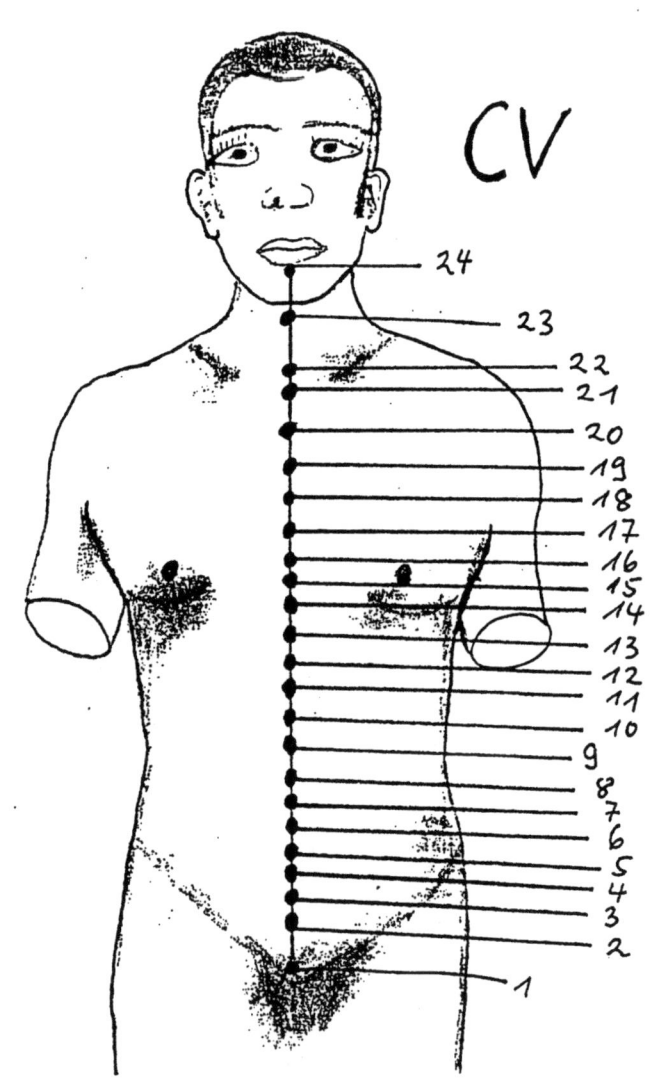

CV

24
23
22
21
20
19
18
17
16
15
14
13
12
11
10
9
8
7
6
5
4
3
2
1

LITERATURE

Essentials of Chinese Acupuncture, Foreign languages Press, Peijing China

Introduction to Acupuncture,A.L.Agrawal,S.P.Marda, Jaypee Brothers,Delhi

Basics of Acupuncture, Stux and Pomeranz, Springer Verlag, New York,London

Clinical Practice of Acupuncture, Acupuncture Foundation of India, Rajpur, Agrawal,Sharma

Textbook of Acupuncture Science,
Acupuncture Foundation of Sri Lanka, Colombo, Yayyasuria

Clinical Acupuncture,Acupuncture Foundation of Sri Lanka, Colombo,Yayyasuria

Theorie and Practice of Scientific Acupuncture, Lake House, Colombo,Yayyasuria

Auriculotherapy, Acupuncture Foundation of Sri Lanka, Colombo,Yayyaveera

Acupuncture, A Comprehensive Text, Shanghai College of Traditional Medicine Eastland Press, Chicago, O´Connor and Benskie

Atharwaweda-Das Wissen von den Zaubersprüchen, F. Rückert, Orient-Buchhandlung, Hannover 1923

Die Dreigestalt des Seins und ihr androgyner Ursprung - Eine Untersuchung zur Kosmosophie des Veda, E. Richter, Bremen 1983

Die Botschaft der Veden, Divyanand 1989

ADDRESSES

Ram Seth Prakash Charitable Hospital,
Department for Acupuncture, Sandila, India U.P.

Acupuncture Clinic, Dr. Ravinder, Shamli, U.P. India

Indian Society of Medical Acupuncturists, Dr. Kapur,
Residence cum Clinic, A 14-2, Rana Pratap Marg,
Delhi 11ooo7

Deutsche Gesellschaft für Akupunktur und Aurikulomedizin
,Connollystr. 14, 8000 München

Deutsche Ärztegesellschaft für Akupunktur,
Raglovichstr. 12, 80637 München

Dr. med. Dietrich Klüber, ENDO-Klinik,
Holstenstr.2, 22767 Hamburg

About the Author

The author was born 1952 in Hamburg as the son of the historian Karl-Werner Klüber and his wife Dr. med. Rose Klüber, being a physician.

Already before his medical studies he developed much interest in all fields of Naturopathy. Though studying without delay he passed the examination for a healing practitioner so that he could already earn his living for his new small family -wife and three children.

Acupuncture has always been Dr. med. Klüber's speciality and he is member of several medical Acupuncture associations including the Indian Society for medical acupuncturists.
During more than 10 years of regular visits to India he gained extensive knowledge of Indian culture and the scope of Acupuncture in India

Since 1979 Dr. Klüber works at the ENDO-Klinik, a specialized hospital for arthroalloplasty with worldwide reknown and since 1990 apart from his surgical work he is advisor for the Department of Medical Documentation and Evaluation with several scientific publications in this field of medicine.